# SEX, VIOLENCE, AND JUSTICE

# SEX VIOLENCE & JUSTICE

Contraception and the Catholic Church

ALINE H. KALBIAN

GEORGETOWN UNIVERSITY PRESS
Washington, DC

Library of Congress Cataloging-in-Publication Data

Kalbian, Aline H., 1954–
    Sex, violence, and justice: contraception and the Catholic Church / Aline H. Kalbian.
        pages cm
    Includes bibliographical references and index.
    ISBN 978-1-62616-048-4 (pbk. : alk. paper)
    1. Contraception—Religious aspects—Catholic Church. I. Title.
HQ766.3.K25   2014
241'.66—dc23

                                                          2013028048

♾ This book is printed on acid-free paper meeting the requirements of the American National Standard for Permanence in Paper for Printed Library Materials.

15   14      9  8  7  6  5  4  3  2   First printing

Printed in the United States of America

*For Bob and Eva Claire*

# CONTENTS

# PREFACE

MONG MY FAMILY's most prized possessions is a photograph of my mother clutching the hands of Pope Paul VI. Her face, framed by a black mantilla, is full of emotion as she pleads with him. He listens to her intently. My mother's face is the focus of the photograph, but as you extend outward from her, you notice other members of my family. My father stands calmly to my mother's side, smiling. My brother and I peer through the group of adults. I gaze directly at the camera. I am eight years old in this photo.

My mother's uncle, an Italian diplomat and good friend of the pope, had arranged a private audience for my family at the Vatican. We stopped in Rome in January 1968 as we were making our way from our home in Jerusalem to our new home in the United States. This was seven months after the Six-Day War between Israel and its Arab neighbors had turned my family's life upside down. Our family's roots in Jerusalem are long-standing. My father's Palestinian-Armenian family had been in the Old City for many generations, as had my mother's Palestinian-Arab family. Both my parents had lost their familial homes and lands in the 1948 conflict, and in the aftermath of the Six-Day War they decided that it was time to move their family away from this war-torn part of the world. They looked to America, as had many immigrants and refugees before them, with the hope that they could find peace and security and a world of great opportunities for their children. We stopped in Rome to pick up my grandmother, who was staying there with her two sisters. My mother had wanted the private audience with the pope so that she could tell him in person about the suffering of Christians in Palestine and about the threats to Christian holy sites. As important as this visit is in my family's narrative history, I do not think any of us have ever considered it in terms of its relation to the history of Catholicism in the twentieth century. It was not until I began teaching and writing about Catholic sexual ethics that the timing of my family's visit with Pope Paul VI became interesting to me. I realized that we had met him almost exactly six months before he issued his most famous encyclical letter, *Humanae vitae*—a document that restated and clarified the Church's position on artificial contraception.

I have been bemused by that realization for many years now. I like to tell my students about how I met Pope Paul VI and about the photo that my family cherishes so deeply. I joke with them about wishing that I had had the foresight to ask the pope some questions about the encyclical and about the series of events that led to its issuance; it could have really helped clarify some of my research! But in writing this book, I have come to think about this photograph and the meeting it captures more seriously. They are a reminder to me of the perils of engaging in any study of religious ethics. In the photo I am an onlooker, but one deeply involved in the scene as I take in the gravity of my family's meeting with the pope. I am witnessing a moment that is intensely personal, yet also political and social. In a similar way, I approach the topic at the center of this study, the Catholic Church and contraception, as an engaged onlooker who is deeply aware of the overlap of the personal, political, and social issues that inform my analysis. I take these as postures that are necessary for the task of studying traditions of religious thought about ethics and morality.

I begin this book with this personal anecdote about Pope Paul VI because he and the encyclical letter he penned are the necessary starting points to any study of contemporary Catholic teaching on contraception. Indeed, some see his encyclical as both a starting point and an ending. They claim that the definitive condemnation of artificial contraception in the encyclical essentially shut down any further conversation or development in Catholic circles. The idea for this project came from my initially incredulous response to this claim. I could not believe that conversations in a living tradition ever completely cease. Indeed, I see moral traditions as embodiments of ongoing conversations, both internal ones and ones with the broader cultures surrounding the tradition. As I thought further about this, I came to see that though the official Catholic position on contraception has remained consistent since 1968, the issues and cases that perplex our society about responsible contraceptive practices have changed dramatically. Moreover, the discourse of the Church, even in its official manifestations, has also been transformed in significant ways. This book grows out of an interest in these changes and in what they can tell us more generally about moral traditions. It is shaped by my view that moral traditions are at their very core ongoing conversations about complex matters that concern individual persons, as well as larger social units such as family, community, nation, and globe.

In chapter 1, I elaborate the methodological concerns that my project addresses by situating my project within the context of scholarship in religious ethics. Chapter 2 offers a sweeping history of Catholic teaching on contraception that, though not comprehensive, identifies the range of justificatory strategies used in official Catholic discourse. In particular, I demonstrate how these strategies reinforce three different frameworks—sex, violence, and justice—for categorizing opposition to artificial contraception. Following this historical background, I frame my analysis in each of the subsequent chapters in terms of these three frameworks. Chapter 3 provides a detailed discussion of the use of condoms as prevention in the context of the HIV/AIDS epidemic. Official Catholic arguments against the use of condoms in this context are connected almost exclusively to sexual immorality. Thus this case serves as one way to reflect on contraception as a sexual sin. Yet one cannot ignore that harm to bodily integrity and health, and also to the common good, are also important to consider in this case. We see clearly in this chapter how sex, the value of human life, and justice are difficult to separate in the ethics of contraception. In chapter 4, I examine the "morning-after pill," especially the Church's stance toward its use by Catholic hospitals in cases of rape. This particular situation enables us to think of contraception and its relationship to violence. Yet I also attempt to show that sexual immorality and social justice always lurk in the margins of these discussions. Chapter 5 turns the focus to a more global scale and looks at the Church's discourse about population control in light of its prohibition against artificial contraception. Whereas the condoms issue focuses on sexual immorality and the emergency contraception issue on violations against the sanctity of life, this case draws our attention to contraception as an issue of social justice. In this chapter we see that the ethics of contraception is deeply implicated in the discourses of poverty, health care, gender equity, and the environment.

The ideas in this book grew out of many conversations with colleagues and students over the past seven years. It was completed because of the warm and generous community of friends and colleagues that sustains me. I cannot begin to acknowledge each of them. A few individuals have contributed to this project in ways that have been indispensable. Richard Brown at Georgetown University Press has been a friend, colleague, and supporter for many years. It has been a pleasure to work with him and with James Keenan, the editor of this series. They, along with three anonymous reviewers, helped me revise and refine my arguments in this book. A year in Charlottesville at the University of Virginia early in this project helped me get started. James Childress, Marcia Childress, Chuck Mathewes, Jennifer Geddes, Cindy Hoehler-Fatton, Bill May, Margaret Mohrmann, Deborah Healey, Lois Shepherd, and Paul Shepherd welcomed and supported me in various ways through that year. Conversations with John Kelsay about this project at various stages were immensely helpful to me. I am grateful for his friendship and support. Laurel Fulkerson, Martin Kavka, and Amy Koehlinger saved me at my lowest points, and celebrated successes with me. Shannon Dunn, Will Hanley, Rosemary Kellison, Marie-Claire Leman, Carla Reid, and Melanie White all contributed in various ways to this project.

Finally, it is because of my family's support that I am able to pursue what I love to do. My parents Ada and Vicken, my sister Maral and her family, and my brother Haig and his family make my life complete in ways I discover anew each day. I acknowledge their love and support. Of course, those closest to the action—the ones who have experienced every twist and turn of this book—are my husband Bob Cross and my daughter Eva Claire Cross. They make it all worthwhile. I dedicate this book to them.

# CHAPTER 1

# Introduction

IN THIS BOOK I undertake a critical reflection on one religious tradition's response to a particular moral issue: the Catholic Church and its official teaching concerning artificial contraception. It is precisely this type of reflection that I take to be characteristic of the discipline of religious ethics—a discipline that observes and explains what one might refer to as "the procedures of argument by which behaviors are judged legitimate or not."[1] "Procedures of argument" in this sense include the justifications people make to support moral claims, as well as the manner in which they make them; in other words, the term encompasses both the form and content of the arguments. To fully understand these "procedures," one must adequately situate them in their appropriate cultural contexts because, as this study shows, the interaction of traditional norms with cultural forces shapes justifications. It would of course be possible to undertake a more purely philosophical analysis of such justifications—one that attends "exclusively to features of ethical justification qua argument," but doing so would provide a very limited understanding of how moral arguments are made and remade in the context of living traditions.[2] As Jeffrey Stout has pointed out, assessing moral justifications abstracted from their context leads to frustration because what is really necessary for understanding a justification is the ability to understand the "why" questions to which it is responding. Lacking an appreciation of the "conversational context" in which justification happens severely limits our ability to understand and assess it.[3] Put differently, justifications function to legitimate the moral norms and the practices that flow from them within the confines of very particular tradition-based contexts.

The religious ethics framework that informs this study is distinct from a moral and theological one. My analysis of the Catholic positions

1

about contraception is not directed toward mediating or resolving an internal Catholic discussion. Rather, it is directed toward gaining insight about the justificatory and rhetorical moves that a religious tradition makes as it responds to cultural and social forces. Studying these moves requires serious engagement with the sources of a tradition, and it requires, at least to some extent, a reading of these sources on their own terms.[4] Such an approach might leave me open to criticism from several fronts. From the perspective of Catholic moral theologians, my study might appear to sidestep the important issue of whether or not the Magisterium is right about contraception. From the perspective of religious studies, such a reading might appear parochial, of interest only to a limited audience and, even more troubling, as evidence of an underlying sympathy toward the tradition.[5] In other words, one might see my engagement with these procedures of argument on their own terms as tacit approval.

I suggest through this study that this does not need to be the case. In fact, I believe that engaging the internal arguments opens up possibilities for thinking more methodically and productively about how all humans structure and deploy moral arguments. The case of the Catholic Church's persistent opposition to artificial contraception and the challenges posed to it by particular cases is thus an instructive example for many reasons. It allows me to draw two conclusions from this study. The first one is that the official Catholic appeal to three different principles to ground its opposition to artificial contraception reinforces feminist insights about the connections among sex, violence, and justice. And the second conclusion is that the Catholic Church's seemingly unchanging norms and claims rely on justifications that are more fluid, and more revisable, than many would presume. This, I believe, is because communities offer their justifications in contexts that necessarily bump up against a range of social and cultural facts. Most religious traditions frame reasons for their moral positions in ways that are responsive to these facts. This does not mean that the responses conform to these realities, but simply that they take them into some account, either implicitly or explicitly.

In essence, this is a study of these realities and of what happens to official Catholic teaching when it encounters them. In the context of the morality of contraception, the cultural spaces within which the Church and its adherents live out and practice their faith have changed dramatically since the late 1960s, when the Church issued its most explicit opposition to artificial contraception in the encyclical letter *Humanae vitae*.[6] That letter proclaimed the Church's stance in contrast to most other Christian denominations, which were then in the process of altering their positions on contraception by embracing artificial methods of birth control as responsible stewardship of procreative capacity. Much has been written about that encyclical and its cultural milieu. Since then, however, new events and crises, such as the HIV/ AIDS epidemic, have emerged and have affected popular cultural views about sexuality and public health. Scientific advances in birth control have led to new modes of contraceptives, such as the development in the past several decades of oral contraceptives that block pregnancy in the hours immediately after sexual intercourse. Global forces and political realities about population have radically shifted and altered the discourse of international development. The fact that the realities that shape contemporary conversations about contraception have changed reinforces the idea that a simple analysis of the internal Catholic arguments for and against the morality of contraception is not adequate. Although it might result in modest scholarly gains that can help Catholics and others better understand the "procedures of argument," it will fail to notice how the points of contact between the Church and the world around it lead to a diversity of ethical and rhetorical strategies. A recognition of such diversity leads to important insights about moral arguments, especially in the context of religious communities and traditions.

To these ends, I pursue two interrelated tasks in this book. First, as I have already indicated, I analyze one specific example taken from a Catholic context. This is the proximate task of the book, and it requires a detailed internal analysis of Catholic discourse about contraception set against a background of emerging cultural facts. This specific analysis leads to my second, more far-reaching task: to identify and elaborate on significant insights about how communities of religious believers make and support moral claims. Two of these insights are worth mentioning: One is that even the most tradition-bound communities rely on justificatory schemes that are fluid and diverse; the other is that moral issues such as artificial contraception are often difficult to categorize. By pointing to the contested nature of precisely why contraception is a moral problem for Catholics, I discover a great deal generally about how discourses about sexuality, both in the Church and in culture more broadly, are often strongly tied to discourses of violence/harm and social injustice. These ties reveal that matters of sexual ethics are never just about sex; they are also about the vulnerability of the human body and the challenges humans face in trying to maintain just and loving relationships.

I trace the first insight by showing the stark divergence between the Church's response to the HIV/AIDS epidemic and its response to the use of emergency contraception in cases of rape. Both responses occur in the context of a Church that continues to adamantly oppose the use of artificial contraception. Yet in each case, the Church navigates particular cultural terrains in ways that reveal a range of justificatory strategies. I draw the second insight about how the morality of contraception implicates sex, violence, and justice from the official teachings themselves. The Catholic Church, as has been previously noted by the historian John Noonan, relies on different frameworks at different historical moments to support its view. Furthermore, it connects each of these frameworks to one of the Ten Commandments. These commandments neatly correlate with the categories of sexual immorality, acts that harm human life, and acts that promote justice. These insights about the fluidity of Catholic justifications on this issue and about the intricate connections between sex, violence, and justice provide useful information for theorizing more generally about religious ethics, gender, and human sexuality.

Although the second aim is more indirect, it is perhaps more important because it extends the scope of the discussion beyond the Catholic context. I hope to make a convincing case that the morality of artificial contraception is a window onto larger contemporary questions about sex, violence, and justice. Mark Jordan bases the claim that "you cannot understand modern homosexuality unless you understand Catholic homosexuality" on the fact that Western conceptions of homosexuality have been shaped by Catholicism.[7] I think a similar claim can be made about the morality of contraception, an issue that has received minimal attention in contemporary discourse. Catholic ideas about procreation, sex, and marriage have provided the foundation of many Western ideas about marriage. Thus, even as the Church's stances on divorce and contraception distinguish it from other Christian denominations, its impact on larger social ideas continues to be felt. Moreover, because the moral implications of contraceptive practices and attitudes are relevant to such a wide range of disciplines (sexual ethics, bioethics, and public health ethics) without falling squarely into one discipline, it is tempting to obscure these implications. I believe that the three contemporary issues I discuss in this book will serve to refresh our view of the relevance of contraception to broader ideas about sex, violence, and justice.

To accomplish these tasks, I attend to three contexts where the morality of contraceptive use has posed challenges for the Catholic Church in recent history: condoms and HIV/AIDS, emergency contraception in cases of rape, and contraception and population control. These contexts differ significantly from the type of case that was at the heart of the 1960s Catholic conversations about artificial contraception—the case of married couples who wanted to limit family size for personal reasons. The three cases that I explore in this book all clearly and effectively highlight the three frameworks—sex, violence, and justice—and their interrelationships. They also reinforce how Catholic beliefs and practices interact with and influence the broader cultures within which Catholics live. In other words, these examples show us that contraception is not just a private decision but also a deeply social, cultural, and political one, with profound global implications.

## RELIGIOUS ETHICS, NORMATIVE COMMITMENTS, AND FEMINIST INSIGHTS

The tradition of reasoning about contraception, especially as it informs the Church's deliberations on new and emerging situations, provides scholars of religious ethics with one interesting example of how traditions reason about moral problems. As Jeffrey Stout notes, "Because not everyone reasons about ethical topics in exactly the same ways and because any given way of reasoning about ethical topics can change over time, ethical discourse can be a complicated thing to study."[8] Moreover, because of this complexity scholars must delve into the particularities of traditions through either empirical study or comparative study. In both cases, however, what is involved is the identification of particular examples and cases. Stout believes the scholar's normative commitments are visible through the selection of these examples. Quoting Robert Brandom, Stout refers to the "explication and grooming of normative commitments" as central to the activity central to all work in religious ethics—critical reflection.[9]

Stout is right to claim that the study of religious ethics is always tethered to the scholar's normative commitments. Yet his notion of normative commitments is fairly broad, and it is certainly not limited to religious faith commitments. He is simply referring to the values to which one must necessarily appeal in the activity of critical appraisal and reflection. For him these values are most apparent in the selection of examples and the criteria one uses to evaluate and situate those examples. Thus those commitments do not necessarily need to be theological ones if one intends to study religious ethics. In fact, he very deliberately distinguishes *theological ethics* from *religious ethics* precisely because of the nature of the commitments each brings to their study. Thus the theological ethicist is "constrained by duties of fidelity to a theological tradition" and by "assumptions about doctrine and about exemplary texts."[10] The religious ethicist, by contrast, has more freedom; yet this freedom is not absolute.

Diana Fritz Cates agrees with Stout's assessment of the field of religious ethics, but she qualifies it by suggesting a more expansive view of what it means to have religious commitments. Thus, whereas Stout is clear that the modifier "religious" should apply to the subject matter and not the scholar, Cates believes that if one uses the term "religious" to characterize any person who seeks deeper meaning—who is on a quest to understand what lies behind reality—then perhaps anyone seeking to understand a religion's ethical system can be considered religious. She writes: "Those of us who study religious moralities need to be broadly religious in the sense that, during times of study, we are eager to engage in forms of thinking that include (among other things) imagining, questioning, wondering, reasoning, and wrestling, as well as believing and trusting in regard to what is really real and important."[11] Cates, writing about "the living tradition of discourse" on Thomas Aquinas, states it well when she says, "Some people participate from the center of the Catholic tradition, some from the margins, and some from outside the tradition. Some people participate from settled viewpoints, and some from perspectives that are still being worked out."[12] Cates's key insight here is that regardless of one's position, one is a participant in the tradition, construed broadly. The marginal areas to which she refers are in my view the most interesting ones. On the margins, it is possible to combine a feeling of openness to the texts, traditions, and reasoning of the Catholic Church with a more scholarly posture of critical reflection and analysis.

I raise this discussion as a way to introduce my study because I agree with both Stout and Cates that as a scholar I bring a set of normative commitments to bear on my subject matter. Moreover, I believe that sometimes it is important to make these commitments explicit. My reasons for thinking this are not only philosophical but also pragmatic. To put it bluntly, my readers might be tempted to assume that the seriousness with which I evaluate the Catholic tradition signals my sympathies with the tradition. Thus, when my work appears critical of Catholic reasoning about contraception, it might be tempting to interpret it as driven by a liberal Catholic agenda. But this is not the case—at least insofar as I am not interested in arguing for or against the morality of contraception. Nevertheless, my precise position vis-à-vis this tradition and these texts is a complicated one, as I believe is probably the case for most religious ethicists. The most significant influence on the way I read and interpret religious traditions is feminist analysis. I find feminism (defined broadly) helpful for seeing that religious promulgations of moral norms cannot be separated from the elaborate structures of authority that sustain them.

The term "feminist" has become notoriously difficult to define. Indeed, it is a much-misunderstood and -maligned term. Serene Jones, a Protestant theologian, defines feminism in terms of a shared goal— the struggle against the oppression of women and for their empowerment.[13] This sort of broad definition is echoed by the Catholic theologian Lisa Sowle Cahill, who defines a feminist perspective as "a commitment to equal personal respect and equal social power for women and men."[14] These simple definitions, though useful, do not fully capture how feminism has shaped my worldview and my understanding of the discipline of religious ethics. Beyond noting that women are oppressed—not an insignificant claim—such definitions do not attend to the specific ways in which feminist commitments can and do shape scholarly projects in ways that extend beyond gender analysis. Jones presents her definition in the context of defining what feminist theory has to offer to Christian theological reflection. Cahill is motivated by her desire to put forth a natural law model grounded in Catholic ideals of social justice. In both their projects feminism provides a starting point for theological and ethical reflection. For this reason, perhaps, their definitions are deliberately broad and simple.

The philosopher Margaret Urban Walker's thicker definition of feminism is perhaps more helpful and relevant to my project.[15] She presents her view of what feminism means by identifying certain lessons she has learned from feminism. The first is skepticism "about people's positions to know their and others' social and moral worlds." This skepticism, she believes, comes from feminist theory's incisive analysis of the connection between knowledge and power—epistemology and politics. She claims that the moral structures of social orders "are epistemically orchestrated in elaborate self-preserving ways" that ensure that power and status are ultimately about who knows what and about who gets to decide what is hidden or revealed. She refers to this deliberate distribution of knowledge and power as "epistemic rigging."[16]

Walker's insights about epistemology shape this project to the extent that the Catholic Church, in my view, represents a grand example of this "epistemic rigging." The Church controls knowledge as it puts forth moral justifications for its positions. Jordan, writing about the Catholic position on homosexuality, states that it is not enough simply to correct certain passages in specific documents: "Changing the language without reforming institutional arrangements would be useless, even if it were possible." Jordan describes specific teachings of Catholicism as "deeply embedded" and "intimately connected to old arrangements of institutional power."[17] In particular, official Catholic discourse about contraception—a discourse that implicates women's bodies in very direct and specific ways—rarely takes women's experiences into account. Entrenched ideas about gender are intimately connected to structures of power that exclude women from decision making while romanticizing their roles as mothers and moral stewards. As we shall see in this study, discourses about violence against women are particularly prone to this problem.

The appeal of feminism for Walker is its ability to critically unearth how power is distributed along the lines of gender, race, and class. This inequity in distribution affects the very core of the activity of moral philosophy—knowing and understanding what actual people in actual circumstances do to one another. In other words, it affects how relationships are built in the context of unequal distributions of power. Walker is also deeply skeptical about how moral theories are formed, especially about who gets to form them and propose them as normative for all humans. Walker judges a feminist ethic to be useful because "it puts the *authority* and *credibility* of representative claims about moral life under harsh light, and challenges epistemic and moral authority that is politically engineered and self-reinforcing" (emphasis in the original).[18] The Catholic hierarchy is a prime example of this sort of authority, and many contemporary Catholic theologians have criticized it for its failure to adequately represent the moral experiences of the laity. Indeed, in the post–Vatican II era there continues to be heated debate about whether the council did bring about significant reforms to the authority structures of the Church.[19]

Walker proposes an expressive-collaborative view of morality as an alternative to the theoretical-judicial model that she sees as typical of most twentieth-century Anglo-American moral philosophy (included under this model are utilitarian, contract, neo-Kantian, and rights-based theories). Embracing this alternative entails several tasks for ethics—tasks that are both reflective and normative. Along with feminist theory, she is critical of the Enlightenment-influenced view of the person as a fully autonomous decision maker. She proposes three kinds of reflection: reflective analysis, critical reflection, and fully normative reflection. *Reflective analysis* is an examination of how moral norms are enacted in everyday life; she describes it as finding out "what moral norms are actually like, how they inhere in and are reproduced by inter-actions between people, and how moral orders are concretely embodied in social ones."[20] She also notes that this type of reflective analysis can only occur if "factual researches" are undertaken and then serve as the material that ethicists study.

*Critical reflection* is more specific and precise than reflective analysis. Here the focus is to achieve transparency by testing for the intelligibility and coherence of moral norms. This is ultimately about accountability—about understanding "who gets to do what to whom and who must do what for whom, as well as who has standing to give or to demand accounts." The normative aspect of this type of reflection is that it holds the particular norms or understandings to some "standards of shared intelligibility."[21]

The third type of reflection that Walker identifies is *fully normative reflection*—"the attempt to see whether a particular way to live is, indeed, 'how to live,' at least for human beings in a particular set of historical, cultural, and material circumstances." These three types of reflection cohere with the sentiments expressed by Stout and Cates about the inescapability of normative commitments. Walker's third type—the fully normative reflection—describes the type of constructive theological project that I explicitly avoid in this book. Instead, in this project I embrace the stance of critical reflection. I am interested in the intelligibility of the Catholic discourses about contraception. In particular, I want to ask about this intelligibility from different viewpoints. In defining her expressive-collaborative model of morality, Walker writes that morality is "social negotiation in real time, where members of a community of roughly or largely shared moral beliefs try to refine understanding, extend consensus, and eliminate conflict among themselves."[22] This democratic model is certainly not the one that characterizes the Catholic Church, but it does capture what I believe to be the task of religious ethics. In other words, I see religious ethics as embodying a task of "social negotiation," at least to the extent that it can "refine understanding." Although I personally share Walker's other, more utopian political goals about consensus and peace, this project is more limited. It is important to note that the expressive-collaborative task, as Walker sees it, is not just a theoretical exercise—it also has real political implications. The coherence for which she is aiming is not merely in the individual but also rather in the larger community of citizens. What matters ultimately is the "ability of a community of persons to make a certain kind of stable and shareable sense of themselves within it as they live together."[23] Moreover, this activity of justification must extend beyond each community. As Walker states, "Even the most private parts of our lives require a public justification, where this means shared intelligibility."[24]

To view religious ethics as engaged in the political task of community building might strike some as presumptuous. After all, who really cares what academics have to say about religion? Their analyses are interesting but they rarely have the political clout that motivates true political change. In Saba Mahmood's study of the women's mosque movement in Egypt, she describes the role that feminist theory plays in shaping her project. She identifies two parts to the feminist project—a politically prescriptive part and an analytical one. She suggests that in order to enter into the worlds of her conservative religious subjects, she must abandon, or at least set aside, her desire to change their lives in alignment with a liberal, democratic model. The goal of social change is certainly central to feminist sensibilities; to view feminism simply as a practice of identifying gender injustice would drain it of its power. Mahmood's response to this posed dilemma is interesting. She is not interested in merely reporting what her female subjects do, think, and feel. She very much wants to critique them. But, she writes, "what I do urge is an expansion of a normative understanding of critique" beyond seeing it as the mere demolition of the opponent's position. Instead, a critique ought to leave "open the possibility that we might also be remade in the process of engaging another's worldview."[25] She acknowledges some repugnance and discomfort about the oppressive patriarchal structures that dominate her subjects, but she believes that denouncing these subjects would impede the scholar's ability to understand "what makes these practices powerful and meaningful to the people who practice them."[26]

Unlike Mahmood's ethnographic study, here I focus on the construction of texts, justifications, and moral arguments. I am aware of an important disconnect: that often, Catholic practices of contraception do not seem to cohere with official teaching. Yet I never lose track of the people who are affected by the moral system put forward by the Catholic Church. I believe that contraception is a helpful case to examine because the goods at stake—sexuality, reproduction, and family arrangements—are so vitally important. In other words, beyond the more obvious questions of regulating reproduction, this subject has implications for how societies understand and structure gender, sexual relations, violence, and social justice.

## SCHOLARSHIP ABOUT CATHOLICS AND CONTRACEPTION

John Noonan's comprehensive account *Contraception: A History of Its Treatment by the Catholic Theologians and Canonists* has been the shaping force of much scholarship on Catholicism and contraception.[27] First published in 1966 and then updated and reissued in 1986, it is a history of the Catholic doctrine of contraception. Like all histories it is shaped by the specific agendas and ideas of the author. Foremost in Noonan's case is his belief that Catholic doctrine changes and develops over time. He closes his book with a revealing metaphor: The doctrine of contraception has functioned as a wall built around the norms of procreation, education, life, personality, and love. These five values embody the Catholic teachings about sexuality. But he notes that a wall can be either a bulwark or a prison—that is, it can either serve to defend the values or it can inhibit them. It is clear that Noonan, writing in the mid-1960s in the heat of the controversy about contraception, saw the Catholic prohibition as a prison. Nevertheless, either as a bulwark or a prison, the wall had a pragmatic purpose—in other words, what mattered were the values around which the wall was built. Thus Noonan's account attempts to describe how these values came to be threatened in the history of Christianity by groups as various as the Gnostics, the Manichees, and the Cathars, and how various theologians and canonists responded to those threats. He writes: "Reaction to these movements hostile to all procreation was not the sole reason for the doctrine, but the emphases, sweep, and place of the doctrine issued from these moral combats."[28]

Noonan also argues that the Church's reasoning about contraception has not been monolithic. He identifies three frameworks that he believes theologians and the Magisterium have used to justify their positions: contraception violates nature, contraception violates the good of marriage, and contraception is murder. I develop and extend these three frameworks in this book by showing how each one relates to a distinct commandment from the Decalogue and also to more recent issues related to contraception. Trying to untangle these three frameworks is not an easy task. Thus, though I rely heavily on Noonan's perspective on the history of contraception, I expand his historical project by noting explicitly the complex relationship among sex, the sanctity of life, and justice.

The other significant work of scholarship in this area is Leslie Tentler's *Catholics and Contraception*. Unlike Noonan's broad geographical sweep, Tentler's study focuses on the United States, and she utilizes a greater diversity of sources, including the experiences of Catholic clergy and laity. Her book is important to the present volume for two reasons. First, her concern with how the issue of contraception affected the relationship between clergy and laity reinforces my view about the issues of power and authority that are at the heart of this matter. She relies heavily on pastoral literature to gain insight on the perspectives of both clergy and laity. Although she clearly sees the issue of contraception as connected to the rise of the laity, she also draws interesting and important connections to its role in molding the clergy's attitudes of their role and place in the post–Vatican II Church. Second, her study urges us to see that a history of the practices and attitudes surrounding contraception among the twentieth-century American Catholic community is relevant to understanding the broader secular ethic of that time. She writes: "This Catholic struggle [with contraception and sexual modernity] had meaning not simply for Catholics but for the nation in which they constitute the single largest religious minority." Her point is that as the major Protestant denominations adopted positions approving of birth control, the Catholic Church's continued prohibition gave it a unique "cultural visibility." She writes that "Catholics enjoyed an odd sort of cultural authority in the realm of sex."[29]

Noonan's and Tentler's works are largely descriptive, although there is no denying that they are animated by normative concerns. In Noonan's case, it is to show that Catholic teaching can and does evolve. For Tentler, it is to demonstrate that the crisis brought about by the debates about contraception is central for understanding Catholicism in America. These two works are distinct from other more recent Catholic work that is unequivocally normative. For example, Todd Salzman and Michael Lawler's recent volume *The Sexual Person: Toward a Renewed Catholic Anthropology* proposes revising many of the Catholic norms about sexuality, including the prohibition of contraception. On the basis of their "renewed principle of human sexuality," they argue that "it is *marriage itself* and not *each and every marital act* that is to be open to the transmission of life and parenthood" (emphasis in the original).[30] Their formulation is interesting because it draws on both revisionist moral theology and the work of new natural law theorists like Germain Grisez. They agree with Grisez that married sexual intercourse is a basic human good, but they disagree that it is a good "that can never be instrumentalized for the sake of some other good."[31]

In addition to the explicitly Catholic literature discussed above, some religious ethicists have also taken on the topic of contraception and the Catholic Church for rather different purposes. One is Richard Miller, in his critical analysis of *Humanae vitae*; the other is Elizabeth Bucar, in her discussion of how authoritative clerical pronouncements on contraception create possibilities for new, creative responses from women who see themselves as standing within the tradition of Catholicism. Both Miller's and Bucar's approaches bring interesting insights to bear on how moral arguments are shaped by cultural forces.

Miller writes about *Humanae vitae* in the context of his larger project of developing a moral approach based on practical, case-centered reasoning. He positions this "casuistic" approach over against what he calls "its main rivals on the landscape of moral inquiry today"—applied ethics and narrative ethics. He builds on Stephen Toulmin's and Albert Jonsen's efforts to rehabilitate casuistry as a modern endeavor, but he finds their analysis to be limiting insofar as it fails to fully capture the expansive and interdisciplinary nature of the practical reasoning central to the project of casuistry. Miller's point is to show that casuistry is an integral part of all moral reasoning—something "that we practice in everyday settings" and that requires engagement in a range of scientific, legal, historical, and interpretive inquiries.[32] One case he evaluates in his book is the Catholic teaching on contraception, especially as articulated in Paul VI's encyclical letter *Humanae vitae*. Miller approaches the encyclical through a "psychoanalytical" lens with the idea of calling "attention to the presence of a 'subtext,' a voice murmuring beneath the surface of an argument, discernible at symptomatic points of ambiguity, evasion, or overemphasis." This subtext is something that is usually deeply hidden and requires an unmasking by the interpreter. For Miller, a document like *Humanae vitae* is not a text, "it is rather a concrete performance, a way of pleading, persuading, inciting, and exciting an audience."[33]

In essence, what Miller proposes is to view this document as something that is clearly entrenched in a very particular set of "cultural materials and social processes." He hopes that his more aggressive, probing reading of the text will tell us something important, especially about how both the categories nature and culture are themselves socially constructed. Why deconstruct such a text when its arguments are clearly stated, and continue to have a hold on many Catholics? Miller's answer is to question what motivates this hold. He asks, "Could the encyclical be affirming something else that previous criticisms have missed?"[34] These critics have taken the encyclical at face value and have failed to uncover dimensions of the letter that can be read using Miller's method; namely, they have failed to notice that a patriarchal ideology governs the letter's modes of analysis. Gender is implicated at two central points in the encyclical's argument: in the connection between bodily processes and the natural, and in the connection between sexual immorality and women's vulnerability to being utilized as tools for male pleasure. Miller's point is that though the language of gender is often invisible in the letter, the ideology of gender is on full display. Seeing and acknowledging this ideology "emancipate(s) us from the grip of Paul VI's moral vocabulary" and ultimately enables the social critic to understand what is really going on in the Catholic Church's official documents.

Bucar devotes significantly less time to the topic of contraception, yet her analysis is worth noting. Her overall project is to set out a new method for comparative ethics by looking at religious women's moral discourse in Islam and Catholic Christianity. She wants to show how women negotiate their traditions' authoritative pronouncements, and especially how they innovate and produce new ethical knowledge. She hopes to counter the more common views that see religious women as victims of patriarchy and their agency as essentially nonexistent. She uses case studies of US Catholic and Iranian Shi'i women to introduce her concept of "creative conformity"—"types of actions which confound the theories of autonomy, heteronomy, and theonomy."[35]

Bucar examines John Paul II's 1984 audiences on *Humanae vitae* as part of her study. In particular, she examines how he is able to justify the Catholic permissibility of natural family planning. The pope distinguishes between acts that obstruct nature and those that are established by God as natural, and he argues that natural family planning is an instance of the latter. He finds support for this in that it enacts the important virtue of conjugal chastity. Bucar's analyses of John Paul II's arguments all support her conclusion that "his rhetoric on the subject creates new possible responses."[36] Thus, in a move that is conceptually similar to Miller's, Bucar identifies unintended and heretofore unnoticed aspects of official Catholic discourse on contraception. Although Bucar and Miller deploy different metaphorical frameworks to describe their projects (uncovering/digging more deeply vs. gaps and rhetorical failures that enable openings for change), they both represent examples of the activity of religious ethics.

## THIS BOOK'S ORGANIZATION AND FRAMEWORKS

The subject matter of this book is complicated by conceptual difficulties about how to adequately categorize the ethics of contraception. This problem is largely the result of academia's rigidly constructed disciplinary boundaries, but it is also due to the fact that contraception has implications that extend beyond the personal realm of procreative decision making. Scholarly discussions of contraception can find a home in many disciplines, such as sociology, demographics, political science, economics, history, medicine, and public health. In a related way, from its beginnings official Catholic discourse about contraception has grappled with exactly how to categorize contraception. What norm does an individual violate when she uses an illicit mode of contraception?

Where does artificial contraception fit in with the traditional categories of practical ethics? In one sense, contraception is an issue that is very much about sexual ethics because it involves the question of proper sexual acts and practices. Yet it is also an issue that intersects with the central concerns of bioethics, such as human dominion over bodily processes, and the injunction to avoid harm. Contraception is also often construed as an area of public health, because family planning is connected to concerns about population, justice, and the common good. Posed as an issue of sexual ethics, it becomes a matter of sex and sexual immorality. When viewed through the lens of bioethics, the focus shifts to the proper value of human life and the importance of protecting life from violence and harm. Finally, the public health view places contraception squarely in the realm of justice, turning it into an issue of communal responsibility—of what we owe one another and of what it means to be a community.

These three ways of framing the issue of artificial contraception—sexual immorality, assault on human life, and injustice—help us to see what is really at stake in the Catholic teaching. Sex, violence, and justice are disparate concerns, yet they clearly overlap in important ways. The Catholic justifications against artificial contraception have tended to retain these concerns as distinct. This is evident in the correlation between these issues and the practice in Catholic moral theology of interpreting acts and practices in terms of their adherence to the Ten Commandments.[37] The 1994 *Catechism of the Catholic Church* organizes its treatment of morality along these lines. It discusses contraception under the Sixth Commandment, marking it as a variant of the sin of adultery. In the Catholic context, to commit adultery is to fail in chastity, the virtue that requires the proper channeling of sexual impulses in ways that protect God's created order.[38] Sexual sins involve uncontrolled or incorrectly channeled sexual impulses. Thus the use of contraceptive methods to impede God's purpose for sex is viewed as an immoderate or intemperate use of human sexuality. Although this is the official way that the *Catechism* describes the sin of contraception, we shall see through this study that Catholic sources rely on a range of descriptions.

For example, there are numerous examples in the Catholic literature of connecting the use of contraception to violations of the Fifth Commandment—the prohibition against killing. Earlier historical sources relied on this description mainly because of a lack of adequate knowledge about the biology of reproduction. More recently, the tendency has been to emphasize a connection between contraception and abortion. Pope John Paul II refers to them as both fruits from the same tree, suggesting that their immorality shares some central features.[39] Related to this point are the persistent concerns about whether certain contraceptive techniques and devices can cause abortions; that is, that they actually harm an embryo. Another variant of this view is that even if contraception does not destroy an embryo, it still reflects an anti-life mentality.

Artificial contraception is also sometimes invoked as an issue relevant to the context of social justice and the common good. This is usually in the context of the relationship between contraception and population issues. Although official Catholic statements have addressed population matters in different contexts, their arguments about contraception have tended to downplay population and public health concerns. When they have invoked population, it has usually been either in a defensive position against advocates of population control or to lament the dwindling populations of developing (Western) countries. A different version of the view that contraception is an issue of justice, or at the very least that it has significant social consequences, is Thomas Aquinas's view that contraception is connected to the conservation of the species.[40] Critics of the Catholic position (both Catholic and non-Catholic), however, have been much more likely than the Vatican to talk about contraception as a justice issue. Feminists, for example, are likely to see contraception in the context of gender and reproductive justice.

The 1994 *Catechism* treats social justice in its reflections on the Seventh Commandment—the prohibition against stealing. Humans are commanded to be just and charitable in their care of earthly goods. This involves not only distributive justice but also preferential love for those oppressed by poverty. Framing the issue of artificial contraception as a matter of social justice renders a very different picture of the issue than those provided by sex or violence as frameworks. Instead of sexual immorality or harm to the embryo, communal goods and interests take precedence. In this view the rightness or wrongness of contraception is not merely about sex or about the value and sanctity of human life; it is rather about how to ensure just social arrangements that are sensitive to the intertwined oppressive structures that characterize contemporary culture.

## CATHOLIC MORALITY
## AND THE DECALOGUE

Thomas Aquinas poses an important question in the *Summa Theologiae* that pertains to the relationship between the Decalogue and the natural law. He wants to know "whether all the moral precepts of the Old Law belong to the law of nature."[41] In other words, are the laws that God reveals to humans in scripture also knowable to humans by reason, which is the proper principle of human acts? In the first objection, Aquinas states that "instruction is in contradistinction to the law of nature, since the law of nature is not learned but instilled by natural instinct." Thus, because laws, such as the moral precepts in the Decalogue, appear as instructions from God, it would seem that they are not to be considered natural laws. Aquinas rejects this conclusion. Reason is the "proper principle of human acts," and good morals are those that accord with reason. Thus, because moral precepts concern good morals, Aquinas writes that "it follows of necessity that all the moral precepts belong to the law of nature, but not all in the same way." Some moral precepts are evident to all humans through their reason; other moral precepts require further consideration by wise people, and still others require "divine instruction" because they concern the things of God. The precepts of the Decalogue's second tablet—the ones that concern killing and family relations—absolutely belong in the category of the law of nature because they are things that "the natural reason of every man of its own accord and at once judges to be done or not to be done."[42]

For Aquinas, what God reveals to humans about how they ought to treat one another is congruous with what human reason can discern. The association of the Decalogue with natural law is important for framing moral discussions in Catholicism because it emphasizes the Catholic belief that God's law is reasonable, objective, and knowable to all humans. What this connection with natural law does not do, however, is specify exactly how the norms of the Decalogue are to be applied to specific situations. In an earlier question in the *Summa*, Aquinas addresses this matter. He asks, "Is the natural law the same in all men"?

He bases his response to this question on two distinctions. He first distinguishes speculative from practical reason. The former concerns "necessary things, which cannot be otherwise than they are"; and the latter concerns "contingent matters, about which human actions are concerned." For both types of reason, there is a further distinction between general principles and their proper conclusions. The proper conclusions of speculative reason are true and right in the same way to all persons. The conclusions of practical reason, however, are not always the same. Aquinas allows for the possibility that there might be cases where general principles of natural law might be applied differently with attention to the particularities of a given situation.[43]

The difficulties associated with the proper application of practical reason have been the source of much contention in recent Catholic moral theology. The debates that have resulted about norms and their proper applications all continue to center on law and obligation. Yet this has by no means been the only resource available historically in Catholic moral theology. Indeed, a strong strain in the tradition, represented prominently by Aquinas, has consistently claimed that moral obligations were subordinate to the virtues.[44] Historians of moral theology note that the tradition that develops in the aftermath of the Council of Trent (1545–63) comes to focus on law simply in terms of the Decalogue, with little or no attention to the virtues.[45] The framework of law understood as "an edict of a legislative will and no longer a work of wisdom" colors morality such that reason becomes simply a way to receive the revealed law. As a result, "the Ten Commandments, understood as a code of ethical obligations, provide the primary criteria of judgment and furnish the principal subdivisions of the subject matter."[46] It was in the post-Tridentine period that a "new genre" of legalistic moral theology developed, and it was expressed primarily through the manuals of moral theology. Four features of these manuals are worth noting. First, they were texts designed to train seminarians and thus emphasized the administration of the sacraments. Second, their focus was the resolution of specific cases, which left little room for reflection on more theoretical issues. Third, they were shaped by canon law. And fourth, they were influenced by Aquinas; although as many scholars, including Gallagher, have pointed out, it was often a distorted view of Aquinas that made its way into these manuals.[47] Namely, it was a view held by Aquinas that overemphasized the prominence of law in the moral life at the expense of virtue.

The Ten Commandments served as useful frameworks for discussing a range of sins and misdeeds in the manuals of moral theology. Yet, as Bernard Häring points out, their apodictic nature led to a mistaken view that the commands were directed to individuals understood as distinct from their communities. He writes: "Primarily, the Decalogue concerns the people as a whole; each individual is personally addressed as a member of the people." This sense of community is connected to the covenant with God that forms the basis of the Ten Commandments. Häring continues: "Belonging to the salvific community is the most manifest basis of his personal obligation. Solidarity and personal obligation are united in perfect synthesis. The salvific-social basis determines the individual's place, duties, and rights in the community."[48]

For the purposes of this book, three commandments are of central importance. The Catholic tradition has framed contraception as a violation of the commandments, thou shalt not kill (Fifth Commandment), thou shalt not commit adultery (Sixth Commandment), and thou shalt not steal (Seventh Commandment).[49] Although the first two have been the prominent, all three relate to contraception in the ways I have identified above: as sex, as violence, and as justice. Furthermore, each sheds light on the concerns raised by different aspects of the practice. In order to understand more fully how they are connected to one another and to contraception, we need to examine the larger role of these commandments in Catholic moral theology.

*Thou Shalt Not Kill*

The Fifth Commandment is the grounds both for the negative prohibitions against causing physical harm to another as well as for the positive injunctions to value life. The *Catechism* proclaims: "The deliberate murder of an innocent person is gravely contrary to the dignity of the human being, to the golden rule, and to the holiness of the Creator. The law forbidding it is universally valid: It obliges each and every one, always and everywhere."[50] It treats the Fifth Commandment in three sections: respect for human life, respect for the dignity of persons, and safeguarding peace. Within these sections, issues ranging from abortion and intentional homicide to scandal and respect for bodily integrity show the deep connections between the negative and positive aspects of the commandment. The value of life is connected to important theological beliefs about God's creative, loving, and redemptive actions. In

*Evangelium vitae* John Paul II describes life as follows: "After all, life on earth is not an 'ultimate' but a 'penultimate' reality; even so, it remains a *sacred reality* entrusted to us, to be preserved with a sense of responsibility and brought to perfection in love and in the gift of ourselves to God and to our brothers and sisters" (emphasis in the original). The sanctity of this reality is confirmed for Catholic believers by the incarnation, whereby God became human in Christ and "united himself in some fashion with every human being."[51] This action reveals the dignity and worth of every human person. Moreover, Catholics believe that in the act of sacrificing his Son, God displayed the enormity of his love for humans.

The insight about the value of human life, however, is not knowable only by Catholic believers. Each person, according to Catholic teaching, can "by the light of reason and the hidden action of grace, come to recognize in the natural law written in the heart the sacred value of human life from its very beginning until its end."[52] Thus the commandment prohibiting murder is grounded in both reason and revelation. With respect to its application, it clearly and with little controversy prohibits acts such as homicide. Other actions—such as abortion, euthanasia, and war—present more complex and controversial cases. As noted above in the discussion of Thomas Aquinas and the Decalogue, the issue of specifying general principles for particular situations can lead to the possibility of different conclusions.

The most recent version of the *Catechism* does not make the connection between contraception and this commandment explicit. Abortion is a central issue related to the Fifth Commandment, and in the context of this discussion, the *Catechism* prohibits any intentional and direct harm to human embryos. As we shall see, much of the debate about emergency contraception centers on the matter of whether there is the possibility that an embryo might be harmed. Apart from direct harm to embryos, there has been a traditional link between abortion and contraception insofar as both have been depicted as instances of disrespect for the sanctity of life. For example, the prominent conservative theologian Martin Rhonheimer views the general acceptance of contraception in our culture as leading to dire consequences, such as a toleration of abortion and the embrace of reproductive technologies. Using a slippery-slope-type argument, he claims that once the link between sexuality (love) and procreation (life) is severed, society then becomes insensitive to nascent life and comes to see the unborn as undesirable. He writes:

"When this inseparable unity between love and life is no longer firmly present in the collective conscience of a civilization the basis for the respect due to every human being is severely undermined, and Christians will fail in their task of fostering the 'culture of life' that is part of 'the civilization of love.'"[53]

## Thou Shall Not Commit Adultery

Sexual activity has traditionally been governed by the Sixth Commandment. It is introduced in the *Catechism* alongside a passage from the Gospel of Matthew where Jesus is believed to have said, "You have heard that it was said, 'You shall not commit adultery.' But I say to you that everyone who looks at a woman lustfully has already committed adultery with her in his heart."[54] This passage immediately expands the scope of the commandment to include any immoderate or inappropriate sexual desires along with the specific acts that might flow from them. The commandment is theologically grounded, according to the authors of the *Catechism*, in the belief that God manifests his "loving communion" with the human race by creating humans in his own image, as male and female. The gendered identity of humans is, on this account, their most essential mark. Moreover, God created two distinct genders to be in communion with one another. In particular, he created in them "the *vocation*, and thus the capacity and responsibility, of *love* and communion" (emphasis in the original). Put in more theological terms, the *Catechism* describes sex between a man and woman in marriage as "imitating in the flesh the Creator's generosity and fecundity."[55]

The remainder of the discussion of this commandment is grounded in this deeply theological vision. Among the topics discussed are homosexuality, adultery, divorce, masturbation, incest, rape, chastity, and contraception. All these are described in terms of their relation to the virtue of chastity, which the *Catechism* defines as "the successful integration of sexuality within the person." In the context of marriage, sex must be integrated "in the complete and lifelong mutual gift of a man and a woman."[56] The prohibition of contraception is stated more positively as an injunction to view fertility as a gift and end of marriage. The invocation of the language of ends of marriage is significant. As I describe them later in this book, most historical accounts of Catholic sexual ethics in the twentieth century point to a shift from viewing procreation as the primary end of marriage to viewing it as equal with the end of uniting the couple in love and fidelity.[57] Catholics who favor changes in the official teaching on contraception often point to this shift in language as evidence that the Church has changed its teaching on procreation and that, by logical extension, it also ought to revise its strong prohibition of artificial contraception. One other point worth noting about the *Catechism*'s discussion of contraception is that it describes it as a teaching that "is on the side of life," a point that reinforces the overlap between the Fifth and Sixth Commandments.[58]

As noted above, Martin Rhonheimer's writings on contraception provide evidence of the idea that contraception is somehow connected in Catholic discourse to a violation of the Fifth Commandment. Nevertheless, the primary basis of his argument against artificial contraception is that it is essentially a matter of sexual morality. He writes: "The morality of contraception is not properly framed as a question of artificially interfering with nature, but rather as one regarding how spouses intelligently and virtuously relate to their own bodies, to the body of their partner, and generally to sexuality and its natural dynamics of desire, pleasure, and procreation."[59] He further clarifies this point by stating that "'contracepted' sex is structurally vicious—though in different degrees, depending on circumstances—because contraception has purposely rendered needless a specific sexual and bodily behavior of virtuous self-control informed by procreative responsibility." In other words, a sex act that is driven by a choice to use contraception is not truly a marital act: "In reality it is sex deprived of its specifically marital meaning."[60]

Categorizing the illicit uses of contraception as violations of the Sixth Commandment is certainly not surprising; I suspect most people would think of contraception as unambiguously the purview of sexual morality. What I hope to demonstrate through my discussion in this book is how the official Catholic responses to recent cases can expand our thinking in ways that point to the deep connections among sex, violence, and justice.

## Thou Shall Not Steal

The connection between contraception and the Seventh Commandment, "Thou shall not steal," is not as readily evident as are the connections between contraception and the Fifth and Sixth Commandments. Yet the *Catechism*'s view of the Seventh Commandment is surprisingly capacious: "The Seventh Commandment forbids unjustly taking or keeping the goods of one's neighbor and wronging him in any way with respect to his goods. It commands justice and charity in the care of earthly goods and the fruits of men's labor. For the sake of the common good, it requires respect for the universal destination of goods and respect for the right to private property. Christian life strives to order this world's goods to God and to fraternal charity."[61]

Although addressing the obvious issues of theft and private ownership, the *Catechism* classifies several other issues as also relevant to the Seventh Commandment: promise keeping, reparations for injustice, gambling, slavery, environmental degradation, human work, just wages, and poverty. These issues are at the heart of the tradition of Catholic social teaching, which is premised on the theological belief that justice is connected to love for the neighbor, which in turn is connected to love for God. The *Catechism* describes important virtues that enable persons to adhere to this commandment: temperance (controlling one's attachment to material goods), justice (rendering to our neighbor what he or she is due), and solidarity (imitating Christ's love and sacrifice for others).

The Church has not traditionally characterized contraception explicitly as a matter of justice, but the cases I discuss in what follows all reveal the importance of justice as a governing principle for interpreting the morality of contraception. In the case of condom use and HIV/AIDS, one cannot understand the epidemic fully without a sense of the economic injustices that fuel the spread of the disease among certain populations and in certain geographic regions of the world. The case of emergency contraception and rape highlights the injustices that result from traditions of gender oppression. Yet it is ultimately the case of population and development that points most clearly to the connection between contraception and justice. In the subsequent chapters I offer a detailed discussion of each of these contexts, following a brief historical overview in the next chapter.

## NOTES

1. Kelsay, "Present State of the Comparative Study of Religious Ethics," 592.
2. Stout, "Commitments and Traditions," 235.
3. Ibid.

4. Such an approach is often referred to as "immanent critique." Dan Sabia notes that this approach is best described as "a family of philosophical-hermeneutical practices bearing complex lineage and associations with a wide variety of moral and political projects and thinkers." Yet what they hold in common is a desire to evaluate critically the "practical norms and social practices internal to some society or culture" by means of sources and resources internal to that society or culture. See Sabia, "Defending Immanent Critique." Sabia defends the view that immanent critique can lead to unconventional thinking and social change.

5. There has been a vigorous debate in the field of religious studies about the appropriate relationship of the scholar to the tradition being studied. A recent example of the contentious nature of these questions is evident in the exchange between Russell McCutcheon and Atalia Omer in the pages of the *Journal of the American Academy of Religion*. Omer asserts that her project avoids his critic/caretaker dichotomy by engaging in "a constructive and contextually situated engagement with reframing and re-imagining *actually existing* sociopolitical discourses, in which justice and peace are points of persistence re-negotiation (rather than dictated by a fixed and *a priori telos*)." I find her description of a "complex hybrid of critical caretaking" helpful for situating my project. Omer, "Rejoinder."

6. Paul VI, *Humanae vitae*.

7. Jordan, *Silence of Sodom*, 8.

8. Stout, "Commitments and Traditions," 24.

8. Ibid., 25.

10. Ibid., 27.

11. Cates, *Aquinas*, 30.

12. Ibid., 29.

13. Jones, *Feminist Theory and Christian Theology*, 3.

14. Cahill, *Sex, Gender, and Christian Ethics*, 1.

15. I want to thank Margaret Mohrmann for introducing me to Walker's approach and the students of my feminist ethics seminar at Florida State University in the fall of 2009 for helping me think through its implications for the study of religious ethics. For an excellent analysis of Walker's value for religious ethics, see Kellison, "Responsibility for the Just War."

16. Walker, *Moral Understandings*, 6.

17. Jordan, *Silence of Sodom*, 4.

18. Walker, *Moral Understandings*, 23.

19. For recent discussions about the proper interpretation of Vatican II, see O'Malley, "'Hermeneutic of Reform'"; and Sullivan, "Development in Teaching Authority."

20. Walker, *Moral Understandings*, 11.

21. Ibid., 12.

22. Ibid., 71.

23. Ibid., 82.

24. Ibid., 121.

25. Mahmood, *Politics of Piety*, 36.

26. Ibid., 37.

27. John Noonan participated in the Birth Control Commission. For a description, see McClory, *Turning Point*, esp. 8–17, 68–69.

28. Noonan, *Contraception*, 532.

29. Tentler, *Catholics and Contraception*, 5.

30. Salzman and Lawler, *Sexual Person*, 189.

31. Ibid.

32. Miller, *Casuistry*, 7.

33. Ibid., 130.

34. Ibid., 134.

35. Bucar, *Creative Conformity*, 1.

36. Ibid., 61.

37. This practice dates to the early penitentials, who organized sins in terms of the Decalogue. As Servais Pinckaers has noted, the manuals' focus on the Decalogue is a narrowing of the rich discussion of law in Aquinas. See Pinckaers, *Morality*, 34.

38. For a discussion of the meanings of chastity, see Connery, "Notes," 628. He offers a more "comprehensive definition" of chastity, claiming that it is not just the control of the appetite for sexual pleasure but also "the virtue which moderates the use of the generative faculty."

39. He writes: "Certainly, from the moral point of view contraception and abortion are *specifically different* evils: the former contradicts the full truth of the sexual act as the proper expression of conjugal love, while the latter destroys the life of a human being; the former is opposed to the virtue of chastity in marriage, the latter is opposed to the virtue of justice and directly violates the divine commandment "You shall not kill." But despite their differences of nature and moral gravity, contraception and abortion are often closely connected, as fruits of the same tree." John Paul II, *Gospel of Life*, par. 13.

40. John Noonan provides an excellent analysis of Aquinas's emphasis on the preservation of the species as a "natural good obtained by intercourse." See Noonan, *Contraception*, 244–46.

41. Baumgarth and Regan, *Saint Thomas Aquinas*, STI-II, Q. 100, AA, 1.

42. Ibid.

43. Question 94, article 4 (Baumgarth and Regan, *Saint Thomas Aquinas*, 51).

44. Pinckaers, *Morality*, 32.

45. It is likely that the emphasis on the Ten Commandments that is solidified by the Council of Trent may partly have been a result of the emphasis that the Protestant reformers placed on the Decalogue. John Calvin wrote at length about the commandments, explicating the significance and meaning of each one. In general, though, he viewed the commandments in their written form as God's attempt to give humans a "clearer witness of what was too obscure in the natural law." He also claimed that this direct revelation from God serves to "shake off our listlessness, and strike more vigorously our mind and memory." Calvin, *Institutes of the Christian Religion*, book II, chap. VIII.1.

46. Pinckaers, *Morality*, 34. Pinckaers also notes that manuals include the five commandments of the Church in organizing the subject matter of moral theology. These cover mass attendance, reception of the Eucharist and confession of sins at least once a year, abstaining from meat on Friday, and fasting during lent. Pinckaers, *Morality*, 35.

47. Gallagher, *Time Past, Time Future*, 35.

48. Häring, "Commandments," 7.

49. The Ten Commandments appear in the Bible in two different forms, in Exodus 20:1–17 and in Deuteronomy 5:6–18. The two versions are very similar, with discrepancies over the commandment about the Sabbath and about whether coveting another's wife should constitute a separate sin from coveting a neighbor's property. This has led to two different numbering systems. Cross, *Oxford Dictionary*, 316.

50. *Catechism of the Catholic Church*, pt. III, sec. 2, chap. 1, art. 5, par. 2261.

51. John Paul II, *Gospel of Life*, par. 2.

52. Ibid.

53. Rhonheimer, *Ethics of Procreation*, 38.

54. *Catechism*, art. 6; Mt 5:27–28.

55. *Catechism*, art. 6, par. 2331–35.

56. Ibid., par. 2337.

57. The *Catechism* describes this as "the twofold end of marriage: the good of the spouses themselves and the transmission of life." Ibid., par. 2363.

58. Ibid., par. 2366.

59. Rhonheimer, *Ethics of Procreation*, 35.

60. Ibid., 36.

61. *Catechism*, par. 2401.

# CHAPTER 2

# The History and Grounding of Justifications

A s with the history of any moral doctrine, there are complicated reasons why certain arguments prevail but others fail. Social factors, theological concerns, individual personalities, and ecclesiastical agendas often conspire to favor one particular view. John Noonan describes the history of Catholic teaching about contraception as one of "tension, reaction, option, and development." He asserts that history is a "human process" rather than the "unilateral action of God making His Will increasingly evident."[1] Although Noonan's decidedly theological project does not reject the role of God in history, it does privilege the importance of human interaction with the world. His understanding of history as a human process reflects an important trend in twentieth-century Catholic theology that rejected a static and unchanging worldview and replaced it with a view of reality as historically and socially conditioned.[2]

The emphasis on historical consciousness, advocated by theologians such as Bernard Lonergan and Joseph Fuchs, is a radical challenge to the neo-Scholastic view of natural law as immutable that had gripped Catholic moral theology since the late nineteenth century. Lonergan identifies the crucial distinction between the "classicist" and "historicist" conceptions of the human person, and Fuchs applies it very specifically to the interpretation of moral norms. Fuchs argues that moral norms are open to revision, and that such an openness does not necessarily contradict the natural law foundation of Catholic moral theology. Rather, it calls for a rethinking of natural law. The distinction between classicist and historicist interpretations of moral norms and its implications have now become a staple of revisionist Catholic moral theology.[3]

Fuchs describes it as follows: "The classicist self-understanding of the human person sees the divine *lex aeterna* as inscribed once for all on created human realities, while the historicist self-understanding conceives human reason as a specific and decisive element of the 'human' reality deriving from the Creator, which can and must take responsibility for the human future."[4] In other words, the historically informed position interprets moral norms anew in light of scientific, cultural, and other developments.[5] Though it might be tempting to interpret the historicist view as too willing to conform to cultural changes, the cases I evaluate in this volume demonstrate that the official Church cannot evade the reality of new social developments, especially as they relate to contraception. Indeed, the Church accounts for and responds to the HIV/AIDS epidemic, the morning-after pill, and rapidly changing ideas about population and development. Yet what is at stake is the nature of these responses. How attentive are they to contemporary realities? Which scientific and cultural facts do they account for and privilege?

The fact that moral doctrines exist in reaction and response to "human processes" is significant for my project of situating the Catholic teaching about contraception in broader cultural contexts. Mark Jordan asserts that in the Catholic moral tradition, "there *is* no unified tradition." He continues: "Even when the words remain the same, the contexts around them shift decisively—contexts of definition and argumentation, of purpose and procedure."[6] Noonan's careful historical analysis reveals the historical roots of the threefold classification of contraception's evil as sexual sin, as an act of violence, and as a grave injustice. In the first section of this chapter, I rehearse the key elements of Noonan's historical account as a way to reinforce the notion that complex sets of arguments converge in Catholic reasoning about the morality of contraception. In some places I supplement his account with a fresh look at some of the sources; but for the most part I take Noonan's historical treatment as the basis of the analysis of contraception in this volume.[7] In the second section of the chapter, I turn to the contemporary period, beginning with the events surrounding Pope Paul VI's 1968 encyclical on birth control, *Humanae vitae*—events that transpired after Noonan's study was published. Finally, I attend to the ways that the discourse about contraception has embraced the rhetoric of justice in the post–*Humanae vitae* era. This is evident in the rhetoric of both supporters and opponents of the Church's official position. My primary purpose in this chapter is to provide a historical context for the variety of justifications by which official Catholic discourse frames the morality of contraception.

## RECOUNTING THE HISTORY

Noonan points to a long history of debate about how to categorize the morality of contraception. The primary sources reveal that early Christian thinkers relied on three possible frameworks: (1) that contraception is evil because it violates nature by interfering with the natural order and processes of conception as ordained by God; (2) that contraception is evil because it violates the goods of marriage—especially the primary good, procreation; and (3) that contraception is evil because it constitutes murder.[8] These three frameworks overlap at certain points, yet they each represent a distinct aspect of what Christians have believed is morally at stake when humans deliberately attempt to control procreation. This tripartite scheme is revealing but perhaps not surprising. After all, it is not uncommon for moral traditions to rely on a range of justifications. More surprising about contraception is that moralists have struggled with identifying the precise nature of what is being violated when an agent deliberately attempts to prevent conception. When viewed through the feminist lens I described in the last chapter, contraception as a threefold violation looks interesting for different reasons. It mirrors a line of feminist argument that links sex, violence, and injustice together in a way that has significant implications for how we evaluate moral arguments, especially those that pertain to human sexuality.

### Contraception Is Evil Because It Is a Sin against Nature

The category of sins against nature has an interesting and complex history in Catholic ethics. Mark Jordan notes that "*every* erotic or quasi-erotic act that can be performed by human bodies *except* penile–vaginal intercourse between two partners who are not primarily seeking pleasure and who do not intend to prevent conception" (emphasis in the original) has at one time been deemed a sin against nature.[9] Generally, these acts have been judged as such insofar as they are perceived to be sins against God's created order, and thus offenses against God. Two different versions of this judgment are worth noting. One is that these acts violate the rational nature that is distinctive of humans. The other is that these acts undermine the common good, the ordered state of human community that enables individual humans to flourish. The second version is often obscured and is incorrectly reduced to the first. To do so overlooks an important difference; the first version emphasizes a static view of history and of moral norms, whereas the latter suggests responsiveness and dynamism in the face of challenges to human rationality and the common good.

The Catholic tradition has consistently viewed same-sex sexual acts as the most serious of the sexual vices against nature, but has also included contraception and masturbation in this category. It might seem puzzling to characterize homosexual acts, masturbation, and contraception by married couples as similar types of sins, yet that connection points to what is at stake for Catholic moralists: Impeding the procreative purpose of sexual acts radically transforms the nature of such acts. Of particular importance for the tradition, it is precisely this purpose that gives sexual acts their justification. Thus homosexual acts, masturbation, and marital sexual acts that use contraception are all illicit because they interfere with the procreative potential and purpose of sex.

Thinking about contraception as a violation of the specific purpose of the sexual organs was especially relevant to one specific contraceptive practice—coitus interruptus—the practice of male withdrawal to avoid depositing sperm in the woman's vagina. Many historians believe this practice to be the most ancient and widely used method of contraception, because unlike other methods, it involves no artificial devices of any sort. The morality of this practice has troubled Catholic theologians for several reasons. First is the problem of "spilled seed" and whether willfully destroying sperm could constitute an assault on life. Another reason was that the practice of withdrawal was a clear use of the sexual organs for a purpose other than procreation. In the language of Catholic moral theology, the act did not achieve its finality or intended end. Unlike barrier methods of contraception, interrupting sexual intercourse so that male ejaculation is achieved outside the woman's body means that the sperm is not deposited where it is naturally intended. Expressing the moral harm this way emphasizes a very biological and physical understanding of sexual acts.

In addition to the concern about violating the biological structure of the act, worries about "spilled" or wasted seed have often been connected in Christian discourse to the biblical story of Onan in the Book

of Genesis. Onan was commanded by his father, Judah, to have intercourse with Tamar, his brother Er's wife. According to Genesis, Er was
"wicked in the sight of the Lord and the Lord slew him." Because Er,
Judah's first-born, had not fathered a son, the duty fell on his brother,
Onan, who has intercourse with Tamar, but he "spilled the semen on
the ground, lest he should give offspring to his brother." God slew
Onan as punishment for this act (Gen 38:2–11). Thus, throughout
Christian and Jewish history, scholars have debated the true meaning
of Onan's act. Noonan, however, is quite convinced that the Onan story
on its own did not play a large role in Christian responses to contraception. He writes, "The biblical anecdote influenced, but did not
dominate, the view of contraception: It was usually interpreted as a
condemnation of coitus interruptus, sometimes as condemnation of all
contraception. It was never used alone without reference to the 'unnaturalness' of the behavior which God punished in Onan."[10]

Noonan turns to the writings of Thomas Aquinas in order to explain
more fully the implications of viewing contraception as a sin against
nature. He begins by noting a perceived incoherence in Aquinas's treatment of the sin of contraception and its relationship to other "acts of
lechery." Aquinas famously concludes that acts against nature are more
sinful than other acts of lechery such as adultery, seduction, and rape.
This conclusion strikes modern readers as especially anachronistic.
How could masturbation be more morally reprehensible than rape?
Noonan explains that Aquinas evaluates these two types of acts differently because they reflect a more fundamental distinction between the
natural and the rational order. For Aquinas, the rational order is the
order of right reason and it is distinctive to human animals; it describes
the human capacity to act on the basic precepts of the natural law.
These precepts are to love God and to love the neighbor. The natural
order, by contrast, is "what nature has taught all animals."[11] Aquinas
writes in the *Summa Theologiae*: "Just as the ordering of right reason
proceeds from man, so the order of nature is from God Himself: where-
fore in sins contrary to nature, whereby the very order of nature is violated, an injury is done to God, the ordainer of nature."[12] He is
responding here to the objection that sexual sins that harm the other
such as rape and adultery ought to be viewed as more serious because
they violate neighbor love. Unnatural sins do not injure another and
thus do not violate the norm of neighbor love, but they injure God by

violating his created order. Noonan's point is that for Aquinas, nature is instituted by God and therefore should not be altered by man.

Aquinas and other medieval theologians hold that sexual intercourse was ordained by God to have only one legitimate end: procreation. Noonan notes that Aquinas also addresses the question of whether it was ever lawful to have intercourse for the sake of health. He responds to the objection that "if marital coitus is good, a sufficiently good intention is the purpose of health." Aquinas replies: "Although it is not evil in itself to intend to keep oneself in good health, this intention becomes evil if one intends health by something that is not naturally ordained for that purpose; for instance, if one sought only bodily health by the sacrament of baptism; and the same applies to the act of coitus."[13] This passage reaffirms Aquinas's view that coitus only has one natural and lawful end. Aquinas also addresses the question of the purposes of intercourse in the context of sterile couples. He writes: "If, *per accidens*, generation cannot follow from emission of the seed, this is not against nature, nor a sin, as if it happens that the woman is sterile."[14] In this passage Aquinas affirms that intercourse while pregnant, with the sterile, and with those lacking procreative potential is classified as nonprocreative, but that does not render it unnatural.[15] He notes that these nonprocreative acts still entail the deposit of semen in the vagina—insemination is the act of nature. What is unnatural is when insemination cannot occur.[16] This passage raises a question about the meaning and implications of "procreation" as an end. It appears more accurate to say that insemination is the goal—the depositing of the male sperm in the woman's vagina. Thus, even when procreation is physically impossible, the sexual act must conform to a rigidly delineated structure.

Aquinas solidifies the natural law argument in the context of marriage and sexuality, and it has continued to have great authority for the Catholic hierarchy. One common way to describe the natural law argument about procreative purpose is to phrase it in terms of the natural purposes of bodily organs. This way of using the natural law argument is often referred to in a derogatory way as "physicalism." Charles Curran defines physicalism as "the a priori identification of the human moral act with the physical or biological aspects of the act." Curran is critical of the Magisterium's application of a narrow physicalism primarily to sexual acts. This he sees as a sharp contrast to the moral methodology of magisterial teachings on social issues such as war or the economy, which emphasize context more readily. In fact, it seems that the tradition has not usually identified the moral so directly with the physical. For example, Curran writes: "Killing is a physical act, but not every killing is wrong. Murder is always wrong, but murder is a moral act. Mutilation of the body is a physical term. Not every mutilation of the body is wrong."[17]

One can see the influence of natural law in modern documents on contraception in two papal encyclicals: Pius XI's *Casti connubii* (1931) and Paul VI's *Humanae vitae* (1968). Thirty years separate these two documents; and more important, in the context of Catholic history, one encyclical was issued before Vatican II and the other one after it.[18] In both encyclicals, the authors use the natural law argument in very direct and explicit terms; but they frame and deploy the argument in rather different ways.

Noonan describes Pius XI's encyclical letter as a "synthesis" or "distillation" rather than as history. By this he means that whereas the letter invoked the various Catholic discourses about contraception, "its composers were indifferent to the historical contexts from which their citations came."[19] Two facts about the letter are significant for our discussion. First, its publication coincided with the Anglican Church's decision in 1930 to relax its prohibition against contraception.[20] Second, Pius XI offered both natural law and the common good as the primary justifications for the Catholic Church's prohibition. Early in the letter, Pius XI quotes his predecessor, Pope Leo XIII: "To take away from man the natural and primeval right of marriage, to circumscribe in any way the principal ends of marriage laid down in the beginning by God Himself in the words 'Increase and multiply,' is beyond the power of any human law." This quotation captures the very essence of the natural law argument as it pertains to the purposes of marriage. Marriage is a natural right because it was designed by God for the specific purposes of procreation; it is part of the natural order. Pius XI identifies contraception as one of the vices that he believes is threatening Christian teaching. He asserts the Catholic doctrine as follows: "But no reason, however grave, may be put forward by which anything intrinsically against nature may become conformable to nature and morally good. Because, therefore, the conjugal act is destined primarily by nature for the begetting of children, those who in exercising it deliberately frustrate its natural power and purpose sin against nature and commit a deed which is shameful and intrinsically vicious."[21] He is never specific, however, about how the concept of nature is functioning in his argument. Earlier in the encyclical, he connects the natural with God's creative act, thus infusing the natural with the supernatural. In other words, what is natural about marriage is that it was instituted by God, the author of nature. Nevertheless, humans participate with God to make each individual marriage a reality. Pius XI describes it as follows: "Therefore, the sacred partnership of true marriage is constituted both by the will of God and the will of man. From God comes the very institution of marriage, the ends for which it was instituted, the laws that govern it, the blessings that flow from it; while man . . . becomes, with the help and cooperation of God, the author of each particular marriage."[22]

Pius XI's encyclical letter favors the version of natural law reasoning that evaluates moral acts on the basis of their offensiveness to God. Contraception is wrong because it is an instance of humans exerting undue power over natural processes that were ordained by God. Nevertheless, he does allow for human power, in that each individual marriage is enacted by human reason. Humans are capable of rationally choosing the institution of marriage and of being able to discern its appropriate purposes.

Pope Paul VI is more explicit in *Humanae vitae* about the direct connection between nature understood as biological processes and the laws that govern morality. He writes that "human intellect discovers in the power of giving life biological laws which are part of the human person."[23] This natural law is "inscribed in the very being of man and woman."[24] Human reason is able to discern moral norms by reflecting on the created purpose of sexual organs. This clearly reflects the type of natural law reasoning that has been called "physicalism" by certain critics of the Magisterium.

In another passage about natural law, Paul VI claims that the norms of marriage are constituted by God's design and that using contraceptives to impede reproduction is a way that humans assert more dominion over their bodies than they in fact possess. He writes, "Just as man does not have unlimited dominion over his body in general, so also, and with more particular reason, he has no such dominion over his specifically sexual faculties, for these are concerned by their very nature with the generation of life, of which God is the source."[25] In this passage, the pope is clear that in using contraceptives, humans overstep their bounds. Jean Porter interprets Paul VI's use of natural law in *Humanae vitae* as very different from the scholastic version of natural law. For the former, the appeal is rational analysis; for the latter, it is theological reflection. The scholastic view of natural law, according to Porter, is based in an understanding of the natural purposes of sexuality and marriage "as these are revealed through theological reflection." The appeal to natural law in *Humanae vitae* privileges rational analysis wherein the physical structure of the sexual act is what reveals its purposes.[26]

Although I agree with Porter's analysis that *Humanae vitae* depicts a different and perhaps less explicitly theological view of the natural law, I still think that it is clear in these two papal documents that the natural law framework presumes certain theological beliefs about God's creation of a specified moral order and about the crippling effects of human finitude and sinfulness. Accordingly, acts of contraception are deemed inappropriate because they interfere with the procreative purpose of the sexual act—a purpose ordained by God. Because this purpose is part of God's created order, acting against it violates the natural moral order and offends God. In essence, the specific purpose of sexual organs becomes the basis for determining the morality of their use. This emphasis on procreative purpose not only grounds this framework; it also informs the frameworks discussed in the next two sections. Yet we shall also see that the natural law preoccupation with the proper purposes of sexual intercourse has an even greater influence on the view that contraception is a sexual violation.

### "Limiting Sexual Promiscuity"

The insistence on procreative purpose was deeply tied to Christian worries about the power of sexual desire and its potential to lead humans to sexual excess. These worries about desire and about promiscuity shape a slightly different framework for characterizing contraception. It is a framework that shifts the focus from nature and turns it inward toward the virtue of chastity, while also remaining tied to ideas about what is natural. Scholars have attributed these worries about the consuming power of sexual desire to several causes, most having to do with local influences on the formation of early Christianity. In fact, many of the early Christian ideas about the role of sex in marriage came about as direct responses to heretical sects that challenged Christian ideals about the goodness of the body and marriage. The New Testament presents two seemingly different views of marriage. In one sense, marriage is viewed as good and as ordained by God (Mk 10:7–8, Mt 19:4–6); in another, it is viewed as a distraction to the Christian task of preparing for the Kingdom of God (1 Cor 7:32–34). Nevertheless, even the support of the goodness of marriage as instituted by God at creation is tempered by concerns that sexual excesses in marriage could detract from God's purpose. In this view nonprocreative sex was a wanton abuse of God's intention for human sexual acts. Thus, in order to protect from inordinate desire and excessive pleasure, that is to keep the will chaste, the early fathers insisted on procreation as a requirement of sexual intercourse. Clement of Alexandria, the influential second-century Church father, writes: "A man who marries for the sake of begetting children must practice continence so that it is not desire he feels for his wife, whom he ought to love, and so that he may beget children with a chaste and controlled will."[27]

Clement is not alone in his view that intercourse when "fruitful insemination" is impossible is seriously sinful. Along with Origen and others, he claims that the primary purpose of sex must be procreation. Yet as Noonan shows, a minority of important early Christian thinkers, such as Lactantius and Saint John Chrysostom, believe that intercourse in marriage has another purpose. Relying on Paul's discussion in Corinthians, which claims that marriage is a remedy for incontinence, these ancient authors articulate a slightly expanded, although not altogether positive, view of sex. Thus, Chrysostom teaches, "there are two reasons why marriage was instituted, that we may live chastely and that we may become parents."[28] Marriage is a way to ensure that human sexual desire is properly channeled. Although this passage still appears to privilege procreation as a primary purpose, it does acknowledge that marriage serves to satisfy sexual desire.

As stated above, the attempts to resolve some of these tensions about sex in marriage were shaped by challenges from heretical sects. Most significant for Catholic ethics was the battle against the Manicheans in the third and fourth centuries. It was in the context of distinguishing themselves from the Manicheans that Christian theologians solidified their opposition to contraception, while also affirming the goodness of sexuality. The Manicheans' views against procreative sex and against the goodness of human creation incited strong reactions from fourth-century Christians, who asserted that human creation was good; hence sex for procreative purposes was as well. The most prominent of these was Saint Augustine of Hippo, whose writings on marriage and sexuality played an influential role in the development of Christian sexual ethics. Although Augustine continues to affirm procreation as a primary purpose of sex, his own experiences with sex and contraception contributed to his worries about the connection between contraception and sexual excess.

Augustine's life, especially as recounted by him in his *Confessions*, is the source of endless speculation about the influence of his own sexual practices on his Christian writings about sexual morality. In the *Confessions*, he writes that "to me it was sweet to love and to be loved, the more so if I could also enjoy the body of the beloved. I therefore polluted the spring water of friendship with the filth of concupiscence. I muddied its clear stream by the hell of lust."[29] Such passages illustrate his torment over his own strong sexual desires, and it seems likely that such experiences shaped his views about contraception and concupiscence.

In the *Confessions*, Augustine writes candidly about his relationships with women, especially with the woman to whom he remained faithful for most of his adult life. He contrasts their relationship to a proper, lawful marriage: "She was not my partner in what is called lawful marriage. I had found her in my state of wandering desire and lack of prudence. Nevertheless, she was the only girl for me, and I was faithful to her. With her I learnt by direct experience how wide a difference there is between the partnership of marriage entered into for the sake of having a family and the mutual consent of those whose love is a matter of physical sex, and for whom the birth of a child is contrary to their intention—even though, if offspring arrive, they compel their parents to love them."[30] Later, he again stresses that his relationship was not based on the primary purpose of marriage—having and raising children. Rather, he writes, "To a large extent what held me captive and tortured me was the habit of satisfying with vehement intensity an insatiable sexual desire."[31] In his later years, following his conversion to Christianity, his reflections on marriage and sexuality are plagued by the view that sexual intercourse is a problem, even in the context of marriage. As Noonan describes it, "If marital intercourse was tolerable at all—and it must be if the Manichees were wrong—there must be some good, some purpose, some reason external to the marital act."[32] Augustine turns to the earlier Stoic analysis of marriage to conclude that the procreative purpose of marriage is the only way to save sexual intercourse from the bonds of lust.[33]

One of the best-known elements of Augustine's theology of marriage is his articulation of the threefold purposes of marriage—*proles*, *fides*, *sacramentum*—usually translated as children, fidelity, and sacrament. This theology of marriage, combined with Augustine's views on concupiscence, influenced the doctrine of contraception, but only indirectly. Although Augustine develops his ideas about marriage and sex in numerous writings, his direct discussions of contraception are few. However, one passage concerning artificial contraception by a married couple leaves little doubt about the strength of his convictions on this matter. In forceful and unequivocal language, he identifies several different actions and ascribes different levels of fault to each. The first is "not to lie except with the sole will of generating," and this, in his view, is totally acceptable. Second is "to seek the pleasure of the flesh in lying, although within the limits of marriage." This, he asserts, is a venial sin, as long as the couple is not deliberately obstructing procreation. Finally, those who obstruct procreation through either prayers or deeds are not really husband and wife. They are not, in his words, "joined in matrimony, but in seduction—either the wife is in a fashion the harlot of her husband or he is an adulterer with his own wife."[34]

Noonan reminds us that this passage, referred to as the *Aliquando*, "was to become the medieval locus classicus on contraception."[35] Nevertheless, he also notes that it leaves many important questions unanswered. For example, it is difficult to discern from Augustine's words whether he was only condemning isolated acts of contraception, or the practice. Noonan also points out that although Augustine mentions abortion and infanticide, he is careful to distinguish them from contraception, thus distancing his view from that of Jerome and Chrysostom, who insist on viewing contraception as homicide.[36] Nevertheless, the connection between abortion and contraception is strengthened through Augustine's insistence that both acts are violations of the marriage bond insofar as they both reduce "married partners to the status of fornicators and adulterers."[37]

Augustine only discusses contraception directly in one other passage—as part of his response to an inquiry by Pollentius in 419. His response concerns the general question of remarriage after divorce, but in it he makes clear that it is immoral to have sex with one's spouse when deliberately avoiding conception. He refers to intercourse between spouses when "the conception of offspring is avoided" as "unlawful and shameful."[38] Thus, couples who have intercourse with the sole purpose of satisfying their lust are violating the more central purpose of sex—the propagation of offspring. He acknowledges that before the coming of Christ, marriage was better than continence because the propagation of the species was a necessity. In the present Christian era, he argues, things are reversed, so that now continence is superior to marriage. Nevertheless, marriage is "a remedy for the vice of incontinence."[39] He supplements his justifications against contraception by appealing to the biblical story of Onan. This was Onan's sin, he writes, "and the Lord slew him on that account." He continues: "Thus the procreation of children is the primary, natural, legitimate purpose of marriage."[40]

In the modern period, this line of thinking that bases the evil of contraception in sexual immorality has been radically transformed by the personalist shift in Christian ethics. Concern about desire and sexual lust has been replaced with the language of respect for persons. Thus though there is still some suspicion about sexual desire and lust, their evil is framed in terms of the harms that they cause the other, when the other is used merely as a means to experience pleasure. Pope John Paul II expounds this view in his early, pre-papal writings, where he argues that the primary danger of a contraceptive sexual act is that one is treating the other merely as a means to an end. The change in language, however, does not completely erase the centrality of the Church's concern about misuse of the sexual faculty. Thus, as we shall see in chapter 3 with respect to condom use for the purposes of disease prevention, the official teaching has been shaped by worries that condom distribution implies toleration of promiscuous sexual behaviors.

Interpreting contraception as an issue about the proper use of sex in the context of marriage is, according to Noonan, in part "an outgrowth of a theory of sexual control."[41] As the passages discussed above illuminate, this framework is based on a largely negative view of human sexuality as an activity that must be controlled and limited. It is also worth noting that this second framework carries with it certain presumptions about the stability of gender roles and the role marriage plays in protecting that stability. In short, if the only way to justify sexual desire is to connect it to the primary purpose of marriage, procreation, then impeding this purpose will result in unjustifiable sex acts. This view that links contraception to sexual immorality is also premised on the idea that the primary intention behind contraception is to engage in illicit or "unchaste" sex.

## Protecting and Preserving Life

A very different way to condemn contraception, evident from the earliest period of Christian history, is to say that it harms human life.[42] Noonan notes that this view emerged partly in response to the pagan disregard for nascent life, but also stemmed from the close connection between contraception and abortion that was a prominent feature of that era. Abortion appears to have been prevalent in Roman society, and Christians quickly became outspoken critics of this practice.[43] Their criticism stemmed from the strong Christian regard for life—a regard that led to a view that harming fetuses and infants was morally equivalent to harming adults. It is noteworthy that contraception was usually grouped with abortion and infanticide, which were seen as direct assaults on life and/or nascent life and thus as sinful. Noonan believes that contraception was characterized as parricide or homicide because it could be seen as a small step from considering infanticide and abortion and murder to considering contraception as such. He quotes Tertullian to illustrate this move in Christian discourse: "To prohibit birth is to accelerate homicide, nor does it matter whether one snatches away a soul after birth or disturbs one as it is being born. He is man who is future man, just as all fruit is now in the seed."[44] Noonan deduces that if the injunction to protect life includes all phases of fetal existence, then "it is only one step to extend this protection to the life-giving process."[45] It is worth noting that "the first fairly clear reference to contraception by a Christian writer," the *Elenchos* (*Refutation of All the Heresies*), characterizes contraception as adultery and murder. This was reinforced in the fourth century by Jerome, who in his letter to Eustochium urges her to persevere as a virgin. He catalogues the horrible sins and behaviors of wanton girls in Roman society: "Some even ensure barrenness by the help of potions, murdering human beings before they are fully conceived."[46] For Noonan, Jerome's clear equation of contraception with murder took hold and helped shape Catholic discourse on contraception. Interestingly, Noonan does not think that most of these early Christian thinkers believed that contraception was murder in a literal sense; rather, the process of life-giving, to use Noonan's term, was sacred and thus inviolable. Thus contraception was an assault not on life per se but on the "life-giving process."[47]

Although the biblical story of Onan played an uneven role in shaping Catholic discourse about contraception, interpretations of the "spilled seed" as damaging to life strengthened the connection between contraception and homicide. Noonan's history charts the rather conflicted relationship that theologians had with this narrative. There were times when the story of Onan was rarely mentioned and other times when contraception was referred to directly as "Onanism." Aquinas elaborates on the worry about spilled seed, and particulary about the harm it causes to the species. Though he does not claim that spilling seed is equal to murder, he believes that the potential life in the seed ought to be protected. He writes: "The disordered emission of seed is contrary to the good of the nature, which is the conservation of the species."[48] Clearly, this view about male sperm and its inherent value arose out of incorrect information about human biology. For much of the tradition, theologians based their analyses on the belief that the male sperm contained the entirety of the life-giving material. As Connery notes, "If conception involves nothing more than planting, it does not seem to make much difference whether the seed is destroyed by being planted in sterile soil or removed from fertile soil."[49] Nevertheless, Aquinas's focus on the good of the species suggests a slightly different line of justification. He distinguishes semen from other bodily fluids, because it is the only "discharge" that "has another end in view, since it is emitted for the purpose of generation."[50]

In the medieval period, monks and bishops accepted and codified Jerome's view that contraception was a species of homicide rather than the Augustinian view that contraception was an assault on marriage and a species of sexual immorality. Why this might be the case is not clear. Noonan conjectures that it was either because Jerome connected contraception with potions of sterility, which were a concern because of their association with magic, or that it was difficult to distinguish abortifacients from contraceptives, or that it was a good rhetorical move for scaring Christians.[51] He also believes that although none of the writers from that period make mention of population, one cannot ignore the fact that this was a time of dwindling populations. Thus, it seems likely that demographics would have been an issue.[52] Finally, Noonan reminds us that the Stoic and Patristic emphasis on rationality led to a "hostility to sexual behavior [that lacked] rational justification." This would include sexual acts that were perceived as violations of the natural order, "such as anal or oral intercourse, and coitus interruptus."[53]

Noonan's main observation about the period from 500 to 1100 is that the prohibition of contraception, which up until that point had received varying degrees of support from theologians, became more rigid and, in his word, "ingrained" during this period. This was largely the result of two things: the first official Church legislation in the sixth century against contraception; and the transmission of that legislation over the next several centuries by monks through the penitentials, the handbooks of morality that were intended to assist clerics in the administration of the sacrament of penance. The penitentials presented lists of sins without providing detailed explanations about the moral justifications used to determine the sinfulness of certain acts. Important to note is that the structure of the penitentials was such that actions were categorized according to certain types of sins. It appears that the use of "sterilizing potions" by women is the main mode of contraception discussed in these penitentials. Noonan's careful review of many of these texts leads him to conclude that there is a "close association between abortion and magic, between contraception and magic, and between poison, abortion and contraception."[54] This conclusion is verified by John Connery in his study of the history of abortion in Catholic thought. He identifies numerous instances of official legislation and individual theological reflection that lump together the use of potions of sterility with abortion and infanticide.[55]

In the history of Catholic thought, the view that contraception was homicide has been articulated in different ways. At times it has been described directly as homicide, and at other times it has been referred to as an act that is like homicide. One illustrative example from the sixteenth century is Hostiensis's argument that contraception is "interpretively" homicide. He claims that it is not homicide in the true sense because no one is killed directly; but because its penance is identical to that assigned to homicide, it is similar.[56] Saint Albert objects to the argument that contraception is homicide because they can both be punished by death. He claims that this idea, taken from an exegesis of the biblical story of Onan, is mistaken. Hostiensis argues that because God killed Onan and Er for their act of spilling seed, then one could deduce that God believes that contraception ought to be punished by death. Albert's response is to say that human action—in particular, punishment—should not be based on an omnipotent God's actions.[57]

For the most part, however, few of the great Scholastic theologians embrace the argument that contraception is homicide and choose instead to view at as a sexual sin, along the lines described by Augustine. The most notable exception is the set of arguments that equate contraception with homosexuality or "the sodomitic vice." In the twelfth century, Peter Cantor equated the sin of the Sodomites with the sin of Onan, and claimed that both sins were homicides. Noonan shows how this particular line of thinking influenced the view depicted by Chaucer's parson, who claimed that to prevent conception in marriage was a sin of wrath, not of lechery.[58] As noted above, Aquinas is concerned about the effects of contraception on "the human seed, in which man is in potentiality."[59] However, that concern is framed in terms of the common good of the species rather than in terms of direct harm to the individual. To view contraception as an assault on human life provides a basis to justify the prohibition of contraception as protection of human life. In some ways, this view seems the most anachronistic from our twenty-first-century perspective. We know now that contraceptives such as barrier methods and the pill do not directly harm a living entity. It would seem that the persistent tendency to equate contraception with homicide in the early period of Christianity was tied to the mistaken biological information at the time, which supported a view that the sperm contains the whole of the human being. Thus, deliberately destroying the sperm is akin to murder. Another way to interpret this framework is to note the long-standing association between contraception and abortion—a connection that is not always meant literally but continues to have rhetorical power. Noonan believes that the prevalence of a pagan disregard for embryos and infants provided Christians with adversaries against whom they posited their own normative positions. In other words, the Christian regard for the sanctity of life was tested and challenged by the pagan practices in the early Christian era. In defending the sanctity of life, the lines that separate life from the life-giving process were often blurred. Moreover, the view that contraception was homicide was based on the presupposition that the primary motivation for contraception was an antipathy to life rather than a desire to engage in sexual acts regardless of the consequences. The connection between contraception and murder continues to influence contemporary Catholic attitudes, especially as expressed by the Magisterium. In the chapters that follow, we will see evidence of this connection, especially in the discussion of emergency contraception.

## *HUMANAE VITAE* AND ITS AFTERMATH

As noted above, *Humanae vitae* marks an important moment in the Catholic history of contraception. Never before had the topic been so openly and widely discussed. With the development of new, more effective, and more widely available methods of contraception, the Catholic Church's reasons for opposing contraception appeared to many, especially lay Catholics, as outdated and irrelevant. This appearance was reinforced by the changes in attitudes toward contraception among other Christians. This changed contemporary climate tested the three frameworks that had governed the history of Catholic thought about contraception in important ways. Did it make sense to continue to rely on these as reasons for opposing contraception, or was it necessary to look to new frameworks? Or, as some Catholics argued, was it time to reject the older teaching?[60] The history of the Catholic teaching on contraception from *Humanae vitae* to the present reveals a struggle between a reliance on the justificatory schemes that had supported the Catholic view for centuries and social and cultural contexts that posed new and often perplexing questions about the Church's opposition to contraception.

*Humanae vitae* was issued less than three years after the close of the Second Vatican Council (1962–65), which was characterized by openness to the modern world and a less authoritarian and hierarchical vision of the Church. In fact, the conciliar document *Lumen gentium* (*Dogmatic Constitution of the Church*) explicitly invokes images of the Church as the people of God and devotes a large segment to the role of the laity in the Church.[61] Avery Dulles characterizes the effect of the document as "a radically different vision of the Church, more biblical, more historical, more vital and dynamic."[62] This radical vision had the effect, whether intentional or not, of changing the expectations of many Catholics about how the Church ought to respond to the needs and concerns of the laity.[63] This effect was felt most acutely in their anticipation of Pope Paul VI's pronouncement on contraception in the mid-1960s. Many Catholics felt encouraged by what they saw as significant reversals of earlier magisterial positions in Catholic teaching that emerged from the Second Vatican Council. Most notable in the minds of many was the significant development of doctrine expressed in *Dignitatis humanae personae* (*Declaration on Religious Freedom*), which affirmed the doctrine of religious freedom as a human right and declared that government, whose function it is "to make provision for the common welfare . . . would clearly transgress the limits set to its power were it to presume to direct or inhibit acts that are religious."[64] The attitude of *Dignitatis* reflected a church more open to other religions and to the notion of individual rights. It also represented a clear development of doctrine. For theologians like Noonan, "the promulgation of *Dignitatis personae* was a triumph of development. It showed that development could mean the flat rejection of propositions once taught by the ordinary Magisterium."[65] This led many to ask, if doctrine could, and in some cases, did develop, could the teaching on contraception be revised in light of new scientific and social findings? Whereas many felt that change was inevitable, others held fast to the traditional teachings. The cautious attitude toward change was embodied in the decision to undertake thoroughgoing study and reflection.

Pope John XXIII convened a commission in 1963 to study population, family, and birth. It continued to meet during Pope Paul VI's papacy, even as its membership and scope evolved. The commission was expanded from its original six, all-male, mostly clerical members to include more than forty lay Catholics, including a handful of women.[66] The presence of lay voices, and especially women's voices, marked a departure from conventional Catholic moral theology, which was governed by the all-male church hierarchy. The commission, in a report delivered to the pope in 1966, recommended that the Church amend its position on contraception by allowing for the use of artificial contraception.[67] In light of this recommendation many Catholics were surprised when Pope Paul VI issued *Humanae vitae* on July 25, 1968. The encyclical claims in no uncertain terms that "each and every marriage act must remain open to the transmission of life";[68] and though acknowledging the conclusions of the commission, the pope asserted that the Magisterium could not consider them as definitive because they "departed from the moral teaching on marriage proposed with constant firmness by the teaching authority of the Church."[69]

In the months following *Humanae vitae*'s issuance, theologians, bishops, and lay Catholics expressed their public disagreement with its teaching. The Washington Declaration, signed by more than two hundred theologians, was the most visible of these dissenting statements. It asserts that "the encyclical is not infallible teaching." It applauds the positive evaluation of marriage in the encyclical, but it takes exception to "the ecclesiology implied and the methodology used by Paul VI."[70]

The scope and intensity of dissent to the encyclical letter ushered in a period of great crisis for Catholic moral theology. This crisis centered on the role of individual conscience and the scope of acceptable dissent from Church teachings.

In addition to the issues of authority and dissent, the contraception debate revealed profound disagreements about the proper Catholic approach to the evaluation of moral action, particularly how strongly to weigh intention in such evaluations. In the context of contraception, intention seemed especially pertinent. The grounds on which contraception had been prohibited in the past were tied to a natural law view about the ends of marriage. If the primary end of marital sex ordained by God could only be procreation, then any sexual act that intentionally impeded this outcome violated the natural order of the sexual faculties.

In many ways, the most significant change in Catholic teaching on contraception had already occurred in the 1950s, when Pope Pius XII expressed support for "periodic continence" as a legitimate way for married couples to limit the size of their families. Support for "periodic continence" was essentially support for acts of sexual intercourse that were deliberately intended to be nonprocreative. Couples could intentionally limit the size of their families, but only as long as they did not deliberately interfere with the act of insemination. Thus, deliberately abstaining from sex during fertile periods was deemed acceptable, whereas impeding conception in the course of sexual acts was not. This distinction obviously raises questions about the role of intention in evaluating the morality of contraception. How is a couple that intentionally avoids sexual intercourse during fertile periods as a way to avoid pregnancy engaged in a different act than a couple using a barrier method or the birth control pill, when in both cases the intention appears to be the same? The difference, according to official teaching, is that in the latter case, the sexual act itself is somehow transformed, and not merely by its intention. What really matters is something about the structure of the physical act itself. Intention is of little significance in this evaluation. In the language of Catholic moral theology, it is the act objectively construed that ultimately determines its moral status.[71]

The Birth Control Commission addressed the problem of intention by proposing an expanded vision of the object of the act. It asserted that the "objective criteria for the right choice of methods are the conditions for keeping and fostering the essential values of marriage as a community of fruitful love." These criteria include the following: An action must correspond to the nature of the person considered in her totality; the means that are chosen should have an effectiveness proportionate to the degree of right or necessity of averting a pregnancy; and "the means to be chosen, where several are possible, is that which carries with it the least possible negative element, according to the concrete situation of the couple."[72] Hence, by expanding the objective criteria, the Commission essentially folded in the matter of intention and circumstance into the object and stressed the need for a proportionate response as a way to limit the amount of "physical evil" that might occur.

Many prominent theologians of the time had already been interpreting Vatican II's call for renewal as including a renewal in the way moral actions are evaluated. In particular, these theologians were arguing for a line of reasoning quite similar to what the Commission claimed about the objective criteria of morality. This approach, which came to be labeled proportionalism, was propounded by several important European and American moralists, including the prominent bioethicist and moral theologian Richard McCormick.[73] In *Humanae vitae*, Paul VI explicitly responds to the proportionalist argument when he writes that "to justify conjugal acts made intentionally infecund, one cannot invoke as valid reasons the lesser evil, or the fact that such acts would constitute a whole together with the fecund acts already performed or to follow later, and hence would share in one and the same moral goodness."[74] This passage, which is quoted approvingly by Pope John Paul II in *Veritatis splendor*, captures the essence of the methodological issue at the heart of the contraception debate of the 1960s.[75] The language of "lesser evil" is a direct critique of the proportionalist view that there must be a proportionate relationship between the ends and means. It suggests that the Church cannot countenance any moral evaluations that appear to introduce a form of consequentialist reasoning.

It is also worth noting that the issuance of *Humanae vitae* coincided with a broad shift in the Catholic discourse about human sexuality.[76] In particular, the Vatican II criterion of the "person humanly and adequately considered" challenged a functionalist view of the human body. In response, the language of mutuality and integrity provided Catholic theologians with a way to talk about sexual relations more holistically. As a result, there was a greater sensitivity to the way sexuality affected the human person in his or her totality. Vatican II also affirmed a more substantive development in the teaching on sex and marriage—one that many have interpreted as a significant break from an older Catholic understanding of the purposes and meaning of conjugal sex. Until this historical moment, the Church had been fairly consistent in claiming a clear hierarchy of purposes of marriage. Procreation was deemed the primary end of sex in marriage. Other ends or purposes were acknowledged to varying degrees, but they were always seen as secondary. The 1917 Code of Canon Law, for example, asserted that "the primary end of marriage is the procreation and education of children; its secondary end is mutual help and the allaying of concupiscence."[77] In the Vatican II document *Gaudium et spes*, two passages are worth noting at some length:

> While not making the other purposes of matrimony of less account, the true practice of conjugal love, and the whole meaning of family life which results from it, have this aim: that the couple be ready with stout hearts to cooperate with the love of the Creator and the Savior, who through them will enlarge and enrich His own family day by day. . . .
>
> Marriage to be sure is not instituted solely for procreation. Rather its very nature as an unbreakable compact between persons, and the welfare of the children, both demand that the mutual love of the spouses, too, be embodied in a rightly ordered manner, that it grow and ripen.[78]

Although procreation is central, the authors emphasize the other purposes of marriage. Such openness to the other purposes of conjugal sex raised the hopes of Catholics who felt that it might ground a more open attitude to the use of contraceptives in marriage. In other words, with procreation no longer the sole or primary purpose, couples might use contraceptive means that enabled them to engage in sex solely as an expression of their mutual love.

*Humanae vitae* outlines this renewed, integral vision of marriage and conjugal love through four characteristic "marks and demands of conjugal love." These are that the love is (1) fully human—it is of the senses and the spirit, combining instinct and sentiment with an act of the free will; (2) total—a complete sharing without "undue reservation or selfish calculations"; (3) faithful and exclusive until death; and (4) fecund, in that "it is not exhausted by the communion between husband and wife, but is destined to continue, raising up new lives."[79] Fecundity is one among several other marks of conjugal love that only makes sense when it is integrated with total, human, faithful love. There is thus a shift from a hierarchy that gives the procreative end primacy to a vision of

complementarity that is characterized by the language of the insepara-
bility of the unitive and procreative ends of marriage. There is a rich
and interesting history of this shift; but for our purposes, this shift
serves to mark another way in which the effect of the contraception
debate really extended beyond contraception.[80]

Thus, though it is easy to read *Humanae vitae* simply as an anticontraception document, one must also acknowledge its attempt to depict
marital love as multidimensional. This point about a changed rhetoric
vis-à-vis sexuality has been important for many revisionist theologians.
For example, Patricia Beattie Jung uses the fact of the Church's shift of
teaching away from the primacy of procreation as a way to argue that
its teaching on homosexuality is inconsistent.[81] Nevertheless, despite
this new rhetoric of conjugal love, *Humanae vitae* absolutely rejected
the use of artificial contraceptives, and that ban remains in place today.

## EMBRACING JUSTICE

Although there have been no substantive changes to the Catholic position on contraception over the past several decades, there have been
some changes in both the tone and scope of the teaching and the
responses it has elicited. These changes are not always obvious. However, as Mark Jordan notes, theologians in the history of Catholic moral
theology often support the same positions but argue for them on different grounds. Jordan is critical of a view of the Catholic tradition that
boils it down to "nothing more than a scorecard of votes on narrowly
defined acts that remain the same over time." This view misses the
important ways that diverse principles and rhetoric have shaped the
tradition.[82] In this section I intend to demonstrate how opponents and
supporters of Church teaching have deepened and elaborated their justifications, and to argue that these changes have led to a noticeably
different discourse about contraception—one that will emerge in
greater detail in the chapters that follow. In many ways, these recent
shifts in Catholic conversations about contraception continue to show
the diversity of justificatory strategies available to Catholic moral theology. Nevertheless, what is most noticeable is the strong emergence of a
different framework—one that places contraception more firmly in the
context of concerns about global justice.

In recent decades, many defenders of the magisterial position on artificial contraception have realized that one way to convince Catholics that Church teaching ought to be followed is to provide a new discourse about sexual ethics. John Grabowski argues that *Humanae vitae* relies too heavily on an outdated "morality of obligation" and does not present an adequate account of sexuality and moral growth. In his words, the Church needs to present a vision that is "compelling enough to offer a cogent alternative to dominant cultural visions of sex as merely ecstatic release, personal fulfillment, or a commodity of exchange." Moreover, it must be a vision "shaped and informed by the light of faith to allow people to begin to overcome the disconnect between their experience of sexuality and their lives of faith."[83] In some ways, Grabowski's comments complicate the neat structure I have laid out in this chapter. They reveal the inadequacy of a discourse that depicts contraception merely in terms of how to characterize its evil. Grabowski is calling for a more positive vision, one that provides Catholics with reasons to embrace a noncontraceptive attitude to sexuality.

This deeper and more complete vision of sex had already been put forward by Karol Wojtyla in *Love and Responsibility*, published in 1960. Later, as Pope John Paul II, he developed this into what has come to be termed "the theology of the body." This is a positive vision of sex, which claims that each act must be seen as a total self-gift to the other. More precisely, he argues that each sexual act in marriage must be measured against the principle of respect for persons—to never treat the other person merely as a means to an end. In his view, when a couple uses artificial means of contraception that "decisively preclude the possibility of paternity and maternity, their intentions are thereby diverted from the person and directed to mere enjoyment: 'The person as co-creator of love' disappears and there remains only the 'partner in an erotic experience.' Nothing could be more incompatible with the proper ends of the act of love."[84] In some ways, this quotation mirrors the discourse recounted above of contraception as an act against nature, although the language of nature is noticeably absent.

Wojtyla also explores contraception through the frame of the virtue of justice, and it is here that we see the connection between his view and Aquinas's idea that contraception is an offense against God. In a section titled "Justice to the Creator," he argues that when the members of a married couple engage in sexual intercourse and have "decisively precluded" the possibility of conception, they have committed an injustice against each other and ultimately against God. The injustice against each other stems from his belief that a sexual act where artificial contraception is used is one that leads to viewing the other not as a person but merely as "a partner in erotic experience." The focus of the act is shifted from affirmation of the other's good as a person to an experience of sexual pleasure. Put differently, Wojtyla writes: "Willing acceptance of parenthood serves to break down the reciprocal egoism—behind which lurks the will to exploit the person."[85]

Artificial contraception is also an injustice to the creator because in not treating the other as a whole person, one is not in right relationship to God. Wojtyla elaborates on this point: "When we speak of justice toward God, we are saying that He too is a Personal Being with whom man must have some sort of relationship."[86] More precisely, the proper form of just relationship with God the creator is to recognize the "order of nature" and conform to it one's actions. When a human's conscience is in "harmony with the law of nature," then the human is just toward the Creator.[87] Interestingly, a quotation from Noonan about Aquinas's natural law view of contraception is relevant here as well. He writes: "A norm is postulated consisting in heterosexual, marital coitus, the man above the woman, with insemination resulting. This norm is ordained, its naturalness is established by God. Deliberate departure from the norm is unnatural, a direct offense against God."[88]

Although Wojtyla does rely on the language of the unnaturalness of artificial contraception, he moves away from a reliance on a negative vision that prohibits the act to emphasize the positive elements of conjugal love, which he believes can only be expressed and experienced when a couple does not positively exclude the possibility of conception. As we saw, *Humanae vitae* also mentions these positive elements. But the rhetoric of the Church's teaching since the 1960s, especially in the writings and speeches of John Paul II, has embraced an even more explicitly positive language of sexuality.[89]

We have seen that supporters of *Humanae vitae* developed its position by offering a more robust vision of sex and marriage. Opponents of the encyclical have also shifted their focus. Their initial negative reactions centered on several issues. One was the matter of the conflict between the Church's authority and the individual's conscience. Related to this were matters of infallibility and the proper scope of the Church's teaching authority. More relevant to this discussion, however, was the concern that the encyclical relied on an inadequate account of natural law—one that focused on the physical aspects of the sexual act. Opponents argued that overemphasis on the physical aspects of the sexual act ignored the totality of the person and the couple, and also failed to account for "the historical and evolutionary character of humanity in its finite existence."[90]

More recently, opponents of *Humanae vitae* have grounded their discussions about the morality of contraception in the principle of justice and the ideal of the common good. One illustrative example of the contemporary shift toward justice-focused discourse is seen in the writing of Lisa Sowle Cahill. Writing about the need for refocusing Catholic bioethics, she argues "that bioethics in the twenty-first century must in every case be social ethics, not just as theory but as engagement."[91] She is concerned that Catholic bioethicists "seem to keep getting sidelined by public debates that reduce Catholic moral commitments to the protection of embryos and fetuses"—a tendency that has been reinforced in her view by "the choice of many Catholic bishops in recent years to throw their support behind the rights of the unborn more publicly than behind health care reform."[92] She asserts that a refusal to prioritize health care access as one of the goods necessary for human health is a failure to embody Christ's New Testament mandate to heal and minister to society's outcasts.

The most radical element of Cahill's argument is her claim that simply talking about justice is not sufficient, even for scholars. A commitment to justice necessarily entails taking part "in a global social network of mobilization for change."[93] She provides an example of this global engagement in the context of the AIDS epidemic, where she devotes several pages to discussing the Catholic Church's response to the issue of using condoms to prevent the spread of AIDS. She begins by claiming that AIDS is not a sexual issue, and hence not only about sexual autonomy, but rather is an issue of poverty and sexism, issues of justice.[94] As we shall see in the longer discussion of this matter in chapter 3, this type of move, common to Catholic theologians who support the use of condoms in the prevention of AIDS, is a way of changing the contours of the conversation. The morality of artificial contraception in the context of marriage ultimately rests on beliefs about the nature and purposes of marriage, whereas the issue of contraception in the context of preventing AIDS becomes about fairness and health.

Jean Porter's criticism of *Humanae vitae* offers a further example of justice and the common good as frameworks for thinking about contraception. She situates her discussion of contraception in the context of how contemporary Catholicism can and should appropriate certain elements of scholastic natural law theory. This is a controversial undertaking because she wants to reject the type of natural law approach that Paul VI used in *Humanae vitae* and replace it with a different conception of natural law—one that is more purely focused on theological conceptions of the human good. She argues that *Humanae vitae* was too focused on the physical structure of the act and thus represents a decidedly un-Scholastic application of the natural law. She proposes that an authentic Scholastic natural law would "focus on the proper purposes of sexuality and marriage as these are revealed through theological reflection, and then they [scholastics] judge particular kinds of acts to be unnatural because they are not in accordance with those overall purposes."[95] By criticizing *Humanae vitae*'s version of natural law, she is squarely in line with its earlier critics. However, by tying natural law to theological conceptions of the human good, she expands on those earlier criticisms.

The nature of the Catholic contraception conversation has changed in the decades since *Humanae vitae*, but the actual official teaching remains the same. As I have suggested briefly here, both opponents and supporters of *Humanae vitae* have changed the tone and nature of their justifications. In doing so, they have moved toward justifications that, in principle at least, ought to be less divisive. For example, when proponents of the encyclical foreground the role of sexual desire and fulfillment in marriage, they express a greater sensitivity to the realities of sex and marriage. This sensitivity renders their opposition to artificial contraception less harsh. Similarly, by emphasizing justice and the common good, opponents of *Humanae vitae* invoke a common language that resonates with Catholics, even ones who disagree with them on this issue. What this says about the future of official Catholic views about contraception is beyond the purview of this book.[96] However, in the chapters that follow, I hope to draw out in more detail the finely grained nature of Catholic discourse on contraception by showing what happens when new cultural contexts pose different questions and dilemmas. The three specific issues I examine are related to the use of contraception in contexts different than the traditional case of private marital decisions about family size and the spacing of children. I believe that each of these cases will show us the tension between the three frameworks or categories the Magisterium has used to justify its absolute ban on contraception even more forcefully than the history presented in this chapter has done.

## NOTES

1. Noonan, *Contraception*, 5.

2. See, e.g., Curran, *Catholic Social Teaching*, 54–55. Salzman and Lawler also devote a long section to describing this shift. For their discussion of how this shift affects understandings of gender complementarity, see Salzman and Lawler, *Sexual Person*, 207–9.

3. Curran and Salzman and Lawler provide recent examples of reliance on this view. Also see Gula, *Reason Informed by Faith*, 231–42.

4. Fuchs, *Moral Demands*, 39–40.

5. In the area of sexual ethics, revisionist Catholic theologians have noted that, in recent decades, the Magisterium has applied the "historicist" conception to matters of social teaching (economy, politics, and human rights) while reserving the "classicist" view of moral norms to the realm of human sexuality. More directly, the implications are that social teaching has been allowed to change and develop over time, whereas sexual teachings are seen as unchangeable. See Gudorf, "Encountering the Other."

6. Jordan, *Silence of Sodom*, 65.

7. This chapter is not intended as a comprehensive history of contraception. Rather, I highlight elements of Noonan's account that show the historical formulations and justifications used in traditional Catholic discourses about contraception.

8. Noonan, *Contraception*, 232.

9. Jordan, *Ethics of Sex*, 78.

10. Noonan, *Contraception*, 360.

11. Ibid., 242.

12. Aquinas, *Summa Theologica*, II-II, qq.154, art. 12, ob.1.

13. Aquinas, *On the Sentences*, 4.31.2.2, reply to obj. 4.

14. Aquinas, *Summa Contra Gentiles*, 3.122.

15. Noonan, *Contraception*, 242.

16. Noonan notes that this is why the Church has considered marriages where the husband is impotent as easily nullified—not so with marriages when one partner is sterile because insemination still occurs. See ibid., 289–92.

17. Curran, *Catholic Moral Tradition Today*, 152–53. John Paul II criticized this way of labeling the use of natural law by the Magisterium in the encyclical *Veritatis splendor*. He argues that those who accuse the traditional conception of natural law of physicalism are missing an essential component of Catholic theology: that the person is a unity of body and soul. He describes the natural law (quoting the earlier Vatican document *Donum vitae*) as follows: "Therefore this law cannot

be thought of as simply a set of norms on the biological level; rather it must be defined as the rational order whereby man is called by the Creator to direct and regulate his life and actions and in particular to make use of his own body" (par. 50).

18. Vatican II refers to the Second Vatican Council, which was held from 1962 to 1965. Referred to as an ecumenical council, it was the twenty-first such council in Catholic history. For more information, see O'Malley, *What Happened at Vatican II*.

19. Noonan, *Contraception*, 427.

20. For an account of the Lambeth Conference, see Notare, "Revolution in Christian Morals."

21. Pius XI, *Casti connubii*, par. 54.

22. Ibid., par. 9. Note that he also quotes a passage from Saint Augustine where he invokes the sin of Onan: "Intercourse even with one's legitimate wife is unlawful and wicked where the conception of the offspring is prevented. Onan, the son of Juda, did this and the Lord killed him for it." Ibid., par. 55.

23. Paul VI, *Humanae vitae*, par. 10.

24. Ibid., par. 13.

25. Ibid.

26. Porter, *Natural and Divine Law*, 196–97.

27. Stromata 3.7.58, GCS 15:222–23; quoted by Noonan, *Contraception*, 76.

28. On Those Words of the Apostle, "On Account of Fornication," PG 51:123, quoted by Noonan, *Contraception*, 78.

29. Augustine, *Confessions*, 35.

30. Ibid., 53.

31. Ibid., 107.

32. Noonan, *Contraception*, 127.

33. For different and more nuanced readings of Augustine's views of pleasure and sexuality, see Paul Ramsey, "Human Sexuality." Also see Meilaender, "Sweet Necessities." Meilaender's article is even more relevant to the discussion of contraception. Based on Augustine's views of unfallen sex and his analogies between food and sex, Meilaender believes that interpreting Augustine as saying that pleasure is not a possible good of sex is an incomplete interpretation. Ultimately, Meilaender (himself a Protestant) believes the Catholic doctrine on contraception is mistaken.

34. Augustine, *Marriage and Concupiscence* 1.15.17, quoted by Noonan, *Contraception*, 136.

35. Noonan, *Contraception*, 136.

36. Ibid.

37. Connery, *Abortion*, 55.

38. Saint Augustine, *Treatise on Marriage*, 117.

39. Ibid.

40. Ibid.

41. Noonan, *Contraception*, 85.

42. However, Pius XI draws a very direct connection between these two arguments. He writes, "Every sin committed as regards the offspring becomes in some

way a sin against conjugal faith, since both these blessings are essentially connected." Pius XI, *Casti connubii*, par. 72.

43. Connery situates the opposition of early Christians to abortion in two different contexts. One was an attempt of Christians to distinguish themselves from "a culture where both abortion and infanticide were practiced with frequency, and to a large extent, even condoned." Connery, *Abortion*, 36. Another was a way to reinforce the strength and sincerity of Christian convictions about the sanctity of life. In particular, Connery notes that Athenagoras's explicit condemnation of abortion was in response to charges that Christians were engaged in cannibalistic practices. By showing how strongly Christians valued all life, including fetal life, Athenagoras attempted to silence charges that Christians could possibly engage human sacrifice or cannabilism. Ibid., 37.

44. Tertullian, *Apology* 9.8, CSEL 69:24, quoted by Noonan, *Contraception*, 91.

45. Noonan, *Contraception*, 91.

46. Jerome, *Select Letters of St. Jerome*, 79.

47. Noonan, *Contraception*, 88.

48. Aquinas, *Summa Contra Gentiles*, 3 (122).

49. Connery, *Abortion*, 54.

50. Aquinas, *Summa Contra Gentiles*, 3 (122).

51. Ibid., 144.

52. Riddle also takes seriously the importance of demographics for discerning the prevalence of contraceptive practices in the ancient world. See Riddle, *Contraception and Abortion*, 1–14.

53. Noonan, *Contraception*, 144.

54. Ibid., 158.

55. Connery, *Abortion*, 34–35.

56. Noonan, *Contraception*, 233.

57. Ibid., 234.

58. Ibid., 236.

59. Ibid., 244.

60. See, e.g., Callahan, *Catholic Case for Contraception*.

61. Second Vatican Council, *Lumen gentium*.

62. Dulles, "Church," 10–11.

63. See Odozor's discussion of the ecclesiology of Vatican II for a fuller account of this development. Odozor, *Moral Theology*, 21–27.

64. Second Vatican Council, *Dignitatis humanae*, par. 3.

65. Noonan, *Church That Can and Cannot Change*, 157.

66. However, after appointing such a large number of lay members, Pope Paul VI revoked their power by limiting the vote to the bishops and cardinals and relegating the lay members to the role of consultants. See McClory, *Turning Point*, 96–97.

67. This report is referred to by some as the "majority report" in contrast to what Robert McClory calls the "so-called Minority Report," which was written by the American Jesuit John Ford as a working paper for the commission. According

to McClory, Ford's report was only endorsed by three other theologians. Alfredo Cardinal Ottaviani presented the alternative report to the pope and it served as the basis of *Humanae vitae*'s position. McClory, *Turning Point*, 130.

68. Paul VI, *Humanae vitae*, par. 11.

69. Ibid., par. 6.

70. "Statement by Catholic Theologians," 135–37.

71. For a description of the relationship of object, intention, and circumstance in the evaluation of the morality of human acts, see the *Catechism of the Catholic Church*, pars. 1749–61.

72. McClory, *Turning Point*, 181–82.

73. Some have argued that proportionalism emerged as a way to justify acceptance of contraception. See, e.g., Kaczor, "Proportionalism and the Pill." Bernard Hoose illustrates the complex history that led to the development of proportionalism. He notes that artificial contraception along with abortion, suicide, and divorce provided an impetus for the traction that proportionalism gained in the US context in the 1960s and 1970s. See Hoose, *Proportionalism*, 5–13.

74. Paul VI, *Humanae vitae*, par. 14.

75. John Paul II, *Veritatis splendor*, par. 80. It is interesting to note that the language of intrinsic evil was not used in *Humanae vitae*. The official translation describes deliberately contraceptive acts as "intrinsically dishonest" (par. 14). When John Paul II recaps the teaching of Paul VI, he uses the term "intrinsically immoral." The latin term is *intrinsice inhonestum*.

76. For a good review of these developments, see Selling, "Magisterial Teaching," 93–97.

77. Code of Canon Law, 1013.1.

78. Second Vatican Council, *Gaudium et spes*, par. 50.

79. Paul VI, *Humanae vitae*, par. 9.

80. See Gudorf, "Catholicism," 153–64.

81. Jung, "Call to Wed."

82. Jordan, *Silence of Sodom*, 66. Jordan is addressing a specific historical encounter between Cardinal Cajetan, writing in the sixteenth century, and Thomas Aquinas, writing in the thirteenth century. He notes that while they both condemned homosexuality, they did so on different grounds.

83. Grabowski, *Sex and Virtue*, 22.

84. Wojtyla, *Love and Responsibility*, 234.

85. Ibid., 230.

86. Ibid., 245.

87. Ibid., 247.

88. Noonan, *Church That Can and Cannot Change*, 246.

89. This is also evident in much of the rhetoric of Natural Family Planning (NFP), which not only values sexual experience but also focuses on the positive consequences of chastity in marriage. Indeed, proponents of the NFP movement have focused on the segments of *Humanae vitae* that emphasize the negative effects of contraception on marriage and women. They depict NFP as empowering to

women because it gives them control over their fertility while enabling them to always view the sexual act as open to procreation—as a gift of self. Interestingly, the rhetoric of control that characterizes the NFP movement is intended to counter the view that NFP is backward and unscientific. Proponents of NFP go to great lengths to emphasize its effectiveness as a method of avoiding pregnancy. Its effectiveness is underscored through the use of a more medicalized rhetoric. The attempt is to move away from commonly held impressions of the "rhythm method" as crude, ineffective, and unscientific. See Rubio, "Beyond the Liberal/Conservative Divide on Contraception." For a classic defense of NFP, see Grisez et al., "NFP: Not Contralife."

90. "Statement by Catholic Theologians."

91. Cahill, *Theological Bioethics*, 2. Interestingly, the early months of Pope Francis's papacy reveal a similar attitude.

92. Ibid., 1.

93. Ibid., 3.

94. Moving sexual ethics beyond the realm of personal morality is a central part of Catholic moral theologian Margaret Farley's work; see Farley, *Just Love*.

95. Porter, *Natural and Divine Law*, 197.

96. For more on this point, see Rubio, "Beyond the Liberal/Conservative Divide."

# CHAPTER 3

# SEX

## HIV/AIDS, Condoms, and Sexual Morality

Religious traditions do not hesitate to rethink their moral rules in the social, political, and economic spheres of human life when situations demand it. All too often, however, a taboo morality (bolstered by both religion and culture) holds sway in the sexual sphere, a morality whose power depends on resisting critical examination, thus preventing the transformation of traditional beliefs as well as practices.

—MARGARET FARLEY, Catholic theologian,
"Partnership in Hope"

AIDS is perhaps one of the greatest not only medical, social, religious and moral challenges of our generation, it has forced all of us to rethink and adapt our values, whether we be in governments, business, or other sectors.

—BEN PLUMLEY, director of the UNAIDS Executive Office,
quoted in "Meeting of Catholic Organizations Engaged
in the Response to HIV and AIDS"

HUMANAE VITAE did not address whether or not it is morally legitimate to use condoms for the purposes of disease prevention—at the time, no one was anticipating that issue. The encyclical's focus was on "any action which either before, at the moment of, or after sexual intercourse is specifically intended to prevent procreation—whether as an end or a means."[1] Pope Paul VI was not thinking about whether it was licit to use condoms to prevent sexually transmitted diseases.[2] Rather, he was concerned that permitting the use of contraceptives would fuel sexual excess and immorality, violate God's created order, and harm the institution of marriage. Much has changed since the 1968 letter. Condoms are no longer viewed merely as contraceptives; they have become an accepted part of public health efforts to control the spread of sexually transmitted diseases. In light of this development, how does the Catholic Church apply *Humanae vitae*'s teaching that "each and every marriage act must of necessity retain its intrinsic relationship to the procreation of human life" to the use of condoms for preventing disease?[3] Do the interpreters of Catholic doctrine believe that it is immoral to use condoms to protect from sexually transmitted diseases? Does a change in intention from preventing conception to preventing disease make a difference morally? Although intention is important for the evaluation of moral acts, the Magisterium has insisted that it is the objective nature of the act that ought to matter most. Thus, in this view, even if it is not the agent's intention to prevent conception, the act itself is understood as objectively directed to that end. In other words, the Church judges the means (using artificial contraception, condoms in this case) to be intrinsically evil.[4] For this reason, the Magisterium condemns the use of artificial contraceptives, even in situations that might involve the potential harm to life. For example, the Church officially teaches that the only option for a married woman whose life will be endangered by another pregnancy is to abstain from sex rather than use a contraceptive.[5] It claims that if she uses a contraceptive, she is committing an evil act.

The particular issue at the center of much attention in recent decades has been whether condoms can be a morally licit means for preventing infection from the HIV/AIDS virus, especially in the case of serodiscordant couples.[6] Presumably in such a situation, unlike the case of the woman worried about the dangerous effects of a pregnancy, the intention is not contraceptive—either directly or indirectly—but rather is the prevention of a fatal infection. Nevertheless, since the early days of the AIDS epidemic in the 1980s, official Catholic statements have overwhelmingly asserted that the use of condoms is illicit regardless of the agent's motive or circumstances. The discourse from the Magisterium has also opposed condoms on more pragmatic grounds, arguing that condoms are not an effective means of stemming the tide of the HIV/ AIDS epidemic. How does the Magisterium justify such a conclusion? The answer to that question is not simple. The official Catholic statements appeal to a variety of justifications to ground their opposition to condoms in this context, from concerns about sexual immorality to pragmatic public health concerns about the most effective way to control the epidemic. This variety reinforces my earlier claim about the difficulty of limiting contraception, or for that matter any issue of sexual ethics, to a simple concern about sexual propriety.

Similarly, Catholic theologians who argue in favor of condom use appeal to a range of principles from Catholic moral theology: double effect, toleration, the lesser of two evils. All these principles share an attention to particularity and circumstances and are motivated by a desire to discern a course of action that best promotes the common good. Hence, trying to make sense of the Catholic teaching about condoms and HIV/AIDS reminds us that we cannot understand discourses about sexuality without acknowledging the ways that they are embedded in discourses about violence, harm to others, social justice, and the common good. Such an acknowledgment rejects a view of condom use that reduces it to merely a matter of sexual propriety, which is precisely what the magisterial position does. My point is that concerns about sexual propriety lead the Magisterium to articulate a position that is inconsistent, because it reduces condom use to a mere physical act. It fails to notice how radically different condom use in this context is from other uses of contraception that are driven by an antiprocreative intent. Thus, this example serves to illustrate how anxieties about sexual impropriety and the desire to control sexual acts can overwhelm and obscure contextual and social realities.

After situating the broader cultural context of the AIDS epidemic and the ethical issues it raises, this chapter presents an overview of official Catholic responses to the AIDS epidemic more generally. Most of the chapter attends to the different justifications that the official Catholic responses utilize. These responses illustrate a tension between trying to frame opposition to condoms as a moral issue and framing it as a practical public health issue. Though the official statements reinforce this tension, unofficial discussions on this issue reveal two very different trends.[7] One is a conservative trend characterized by theologians who oppose condoms even more stridently than the Magisterium does. Their conservative argument is characterized by the move of isolating sexual ethics from its social and cultural contexts. This trend is a minority view that is associated mostly with the theologian Germain Grisez. His view of the morality of condom use is certainly not typical of most Catholic theologians; indeed, it is extreme even when compared with the work of another conservative theologian, Father Martin Rhonheimer, whose position on condoms I also address in this section of the chapter. The contrast between Grisez and Rhonheimer serves as a bridge to the second trend, which is exemplified by a wide international coalition of theologians, who foreground the sex–violence–justice nexus and ground their support of condoms in traditional Catholic principles. This trend is exemplified by the work of the Catholic Theological Coalition on HIV/AIDS Prevention, a group founded in the 1990s, whose members include Lisa Sowle Cahill, Jon Fuller, James Keenan, Kevin Kelly, Enda McDonagh, and Robert Vitillo.[8] Their views show that the official anticondom stance is not the only moral position available to the Church. These theologians, along with numerous others, argue that it is possible to support condom use using Catholic principles. Their view has been shaped by ideas about tradition that are very similar to the ones articulated by John Noonan in chapter 2. For example, Fuller and Keenan write: "We do not need to construct an entire new moral system, even at such a critical time as this one. Rather the Catholic tradition is a supple and balanced legacy that we need to recognize, appreciate, and utilize."[9]

It is also worth noting that in addition to the theologians associated with the Catholic Theological Coalition on HIV/AIDS Prevention, some local bishops have also expressed reservations about the official teaching about condoms. In a 2006 statement issued by the Pontifical Council for the Pastoral Care of Migrants and Itinerant People, Archbishop Agostino Marchetto acknowledged the variety of opinions offered by cardinals and bishops on this matter. In particular, he quotes the Southern Africa Bishops' Conference:

> There are couples where one of the parties is living with HIV/AIDS. In these cases there is the real danger that the healthy partner may contract this killer disease. The Church accepts that everyone has the right to defend one's life against mortal danger. This would include using the appropriate means and course of action. Similarly, where one spouse is infected with HIV/AIDS, they must listen to their consciences. They

are the only ones who can choose the appropriate means, in order to defend themselves against infection. Decisions of such an intimate nature should be made by both husband and wife as equal and loving partners.[10]

In addition to this statement, Keenan and Fuller cite several examples of bishops around the world who have recognized and supported the viability of the use of condoms for preventive purposes. As Keenan and Fuller note, "Bishops are able to take these steps because the tradition provides them with a way . . . both to protect existing teaching and to simultaneously engage new problems creatively."[11]

## HIV/AIDS AND ETHICAL ISSUES

The first widely reported case of Acquired Immune Deficiency Syndrome (AIDS) occurred in 1981. Initially, most of the focus was on a targeted patient population consisting of gay men and intravenous drug users. There was also great concern about tainted blood products because several of the early cases of AIDS were of individuals who had contracted the virus through infected blood products. By 1984, the Human Immuno-Deficiency Virus (HIV) had been identified as the cause of AIDS, and by the end of the decade the Food and Drug Administration (FDA) had approved the first generation of drugs that were able to slow down the progress of the disease. During the early years of the epidemic, a majority of those infected died.[12] In the ensuing decades the numbers of people infected with the virus has grown exponentially, from about 8 million in 1990 to approximately 34 million in 2011.[13] Not only have the numbers grown, but the characteristics and geographic locations of the population infected with the disease have changed significantly. In North America, for example, there has been an increase in the number of African American and Hispanic men infected with HIV.[14] On a global scale, one of the most noteworthy developments has been the number of women infected with the disease. Statistics for 2011 indicate that of the estimated 30.7 million adults infected with HIV, 16.7 million are women.[15]

The geography of AIDS has also changed in the past four decades as AIDS has now spread to most corners of the world.[16] The World Health Organization estimated in 2012 that more than two-thirds of

HIV infections in the world were located in Sub-Saharan Africa.[17] Also significant is the availability of effective treatments that enable people to live longer with the disease. In the early 1980s, an AIDS diagnosis meant sure death, whereas by 2012, the prognosis for someone receiving antiretroviral treatments was much improved. Although a cure for HIV/AIDS still eludes us, these treatments have turned the disease into a chronic condition that can be maintained for several decades.[18] There is also recent evidence that the treatments being used to maintain those infected with the disease are effective at reducing the incidence of transmission.[19]

In the early years of the epidemic, a general lack of knowledge about the causes and development of the disease led to some misinformed ethical responses. More knowledge and new effective treatments have dissipated much of the mystery that surrounded the disease. In the early years, Catholic responses were shaped by many of the emerging societal responses to the disease. Kevin Kelly, writing in 1987, identified six groups of issues that reflect some of the earliest ethical concerns about the disease.[20] The first group concerns threats to civil liberties, which include issues such as privacy, access to care, and any instance when individual rights conflict with societal interest. Specific examples include "proposals for mandatory antibody screening, registry of AIDS patients or people at various degrees of risk for AIDS, isolation or quarantine of AIDS patients, laws against homosexuality and drug abuse, and closing of facilities thought to be centers of disease transmission."[21] Kelly notes that though the conflict between individual rights and the public good has existed in previous situations, this disease offers some unique challenges stemming from the nature of the transmission, the social location of most of the victims of the disease, and (at the time of the article) the lack of any effective treatments or cures. Thus, for example, the gay men and drug users who made up the majority of the disease's early victims were already in groups that were stigmatized and marginalized in our society. To curtail their civil liberties for the purpose of protecting society at large required serious justifications.

Kelly labels the second group of ethical issues "scarce resources issues"—what one might call justice or allocation issues. The early years of the disease posed a challenge to certain regions and hospitals, which were suddenly asked to care for large numbers of very sick patients with a disease about which very little was known. Abigail Zuger describes her experiences as an intern at Bellevue Hospital in New York City in the early 1980s, noting the very particular nature of the care that AIDS patients required: "The care is time-consuming and technically sophisticated; it draws on a particular, esoteric, and very rapidly changing body of medical knowledge; the patients are dramatically ill and deteriorate very quickly; their diseases can be palliated but seldom cured; they are, whoever they may be, often difficult patients for physicians to come to terms with; there are infinitesimal risks of catching their disease."[22] This first-person account captures the particular difficulties associated with the early years of the AIDS epidemic, and it highlights Kelly's point about difficult ethical decisions surrounding the allocation of health care resources for AIDS patients.

Kelly identifies the third group as "truth-telling issues" that pit a patient's right to know against a physician's desire to protect a patient. Kelly notes that in the case of AIDS, the swift and severe deterioration of a patient's central nervous system makes it difficult to ascertain whether the patient is truly capable of understanding and incorporating information from the health care provider. Even more significant is whether news of the diagnosis might have negative physiological side effects for the patient.[23] Of course, in the context of an infectious disease, patient responsibility depends on full knowledge of the disease.

Next, Kelly identifies the ethical problems associated with the principle of confidentiality and the associated consequences of discrimination that could result if private health information were to be publicly disseminated. In terms of AIDS, the issue extends beyond the patient's privacy to the realm of information about sexual partners and lifestyles. Kelly also identifies a group of ethical issues that resist categorization. These concern societal attitudes toward the sex and drug practices that make persons more susceptible to infection. He refers to this group of ethical issues as "support of 'immoral' activities." Here, he raises concerns about the use of public funds for "safe sex education," and the distribution of sterile needles to drug addicts. Finally, Kelly suggests that the AIDS epidemic is forcing the field of bioethics to rethink certain end-of-life issues. In particular, he refers to questions about decision-making competence and the complications that homosexual relationships create in terms of surrogate decision making.

Although many of these issues continue to inform responses to AIDS, today's epidemic raises a slightly different set of ethical issues. For example, one central concern is whether HIV drugs are being distributed equitably, especially in the global context.[24] Additionally, more people have come to recognize the roles that gender, race, and socioeconomic status play in the spread of the epidemic, along with how the disease itself reinforces existing oppressive structures. The ethical concerns Kelly outlined are focused on the intimate clinical relationship between physician and patient. More recent analyses of the ethics of AIDS focus on public health concerns about the effects of the disease on entire populations.

The responses of religious groups to the AIDS epidemic have been mixed and inconsistent over time.[25] In the early years, these responses were hampered by the lack of adequate and accurate information about the disease, a situation that has changed in the intervening decades as we have come to know more about the disease. One concern that has shaped many of the religious responses has been the persistent perception of the disease as "a gay disease." Even though most people are now aware that it can be spread through heterosexual contact, religious reactions to the epidemic continue to be affected by moral attitudes about homosexuality.[26] For the Catholic Church, concerns about the sexual practices associated with the transmission of AIDS are balanced against its charitable mission of caring for the sick. A report by the Catholic group Caritas captures this tension: "The Caritas response to HIV and AIDS is grounded in the traditional teaching of the Catholic Church, which mandates the Catholic faithful and Church-related institutions and agencies to read the 'signs of the times' in order to accompany the most vulnerable and marginalized persons found in contemporary society."[27] The reference to "signs of the times" indicates the Church's acknowledgment that its charitable activities do not exist in a vacuum; they must be responsive to the culture around them, and that includes the sexual practices of those infected with HIV. Nevertheless, this quotation also emphasizes that the responsiveness must always remain consistent with the tradition.

Catholic institutions provide much of the care for HIV/AIDS patients and their families worldwide, especially in areas like Sub-Saharan Africa. In 2005, the Church was providing 26.7 percent of HIV/AIDS health care worldwide in the areas of prevention and health education, support for orphans, distribution of food and medicines, and other more traditional forms of care.[28] In Sub-Saharan Africa, this number is even higher.[29] The Church has also been outspoken in urging pharmaceutical companies to reduce the price of antiretroviral medications for developing countries.[30] Although their focus is clearly on the practical matter of how best to serve persons living with HIV/AIDS, Catholic charitable groups also display a concern for the social injustice that is both the root and the consequence of the epidemic. For example, a statement issued jointly by Caritas and the Council of Episcopal Conferences of Latin America (Consejo Episcopal Latinoamericano) states: "In our world that is suffering from HIV/AIDS, the pandemic has been linked in a complex fashion to structural inequalities, to a lack of respect for human dignity, the vulnerability of human rights and power abuse (in particular in relationships between men and women and regarding those who have been marginalized by society)."[31]

## AIDS PREVENTION AND CONDOMS

In spite of its record of care and involvement in the AIDS epidemic, general public perceptions of the Church focus on its anticondom stance, which is viewed by many as harmful. Most public health experts agree that condoms, when used consistently and properly, are a primary and effective means of controlling the spread of the disease, especially when presented alongside other messages (antipromiscuity, profidelity) directed at changing sexual behaviors. The FDA states: "There's no absolute guarantee [of preventing disease transmission] even when you use a condom. But most experts believe that the risk of getting HIV/AIDS and other sexually transmitted diseases can be greatly reduced if a condom is used properly. In other words, sex with condoms isn't totally 'safe sex,' but it is 'less risky' sex."[32] The United Nations Program on HIV/AIDS (UNAIDS) also supports condom promotion in concert with other prevention messages. It noted in 1990 that "the male latex condom is the single, most efficient, available technology to reduce the sexual transmission of HIV and other sexually transmitted infections."[33]

The Church has criticized any public health message that claims that condoms, and only condoms, are the way to stem the tide of the epidemic. As one cleric involved with the group Caritas states: "Regrettably, however, many scientists, HIV prevention educators, and AIDS activists are so fixed on condom promotion that they do not give due attention to the risk avoidance that is possible to achieve through abstinence outside marriage and mutual, lifelong fidelity within marriage."[34] Some Catholic AIDS activists who support the Vatican's anticondom stance frame their opposition as a concern about the ineffectiveness of condom promotion as a public health policy. Thus Michael Czerny states: "Statistics bear out the fact that the wide distribution of condoms as a prevention strategy does not succeed." Yet he acknowledges that if a couple uses a condom consistently and one of them is HIV positive, it "will reduce their chances of infection."[35]

Indeed, the Catholic Church is the most visible resister to the condom message. Yet it is worth noting that it is not alone in its resistance. In Sub-Saharan Africa, for example, the Catholic message against condoms has resonated with traditional African cultural views about sex and procreation. Elizabeth Onjoro Meassick contends that "condoms, in addition to preventing transmission of HIV, also inhibit procreation, which is highly valued and the main reason for marriage in Africa."[36] Along with concerns about how condoms might affect male sexual performance and the experience of pleasure, this is a reminder that the Catholic opposition to condoms is not unique. Meassick's observation suggests that concerns about sexual morality and the meanings and ends of marriage are deeply important to many Africans.

Some are critical of the "condoms as safe sex" campaigns because they perceive them as based on "predominantly Western assumptions and moralities about human sexuality, gender relations, and individual behavior."[37] Katherine Lepani claims that this "discursive epidemiology" is dangerous because it smuggles in moral assumptions that fail to account for "how such information interacts dynamically with diverse and changing cultural beliefs and practices."[38] Thus in many non-Western cultural contexts, the Catholic message that condoms are not a reliable and effective means of HIV prevention aligns with many local cultural views and reinforces them over against the public health officials who communicate what is assumed to be a Western message.

Public health officials have become more attuned to cultural contexts and have also come to realize that simply distributing condoms to at-risk populations is not a sufficient response to the AIDS epidemic.[39] Nevertheless, the public health consensus is that condoms offer a necessary line of defense against infection. The Church, however, continues to be suspicious of prevention efforts that privilege condoms. Their suspicion about the effectiveness of condoms was reinforced several decades ago when Uganda's abstinence-based programs were proving effective. In the mid-1980s Uganda's government undertook an aggressive campaign to educate its citizens about the transmission of HIV/

AIDS. This campaign utilized the ABC (for "abstain, be faithful, condoms") method, which relies on "a tiered approach to prevention that is appropriately calibrated to levels of risk."[40] It allowed for condoms, but only as a last resort. Although the Church embraced the messages of abstinence and fidelity, it opposed any mention of condoms, even as a last resort. A controversy ensued when UNAIDS estimated a 67 percent drop in HIV/AIDS prevalence in Uganda between 1991 and 2001, the years when the ABC prevention campaign was in full swing.[41] Because the campaign endorsed both changes in sexual behavior and condom use, public health officials struggled to interpret the causes of the 67 percent drop. Some also raised questions about the accuracy of the 67 percent figure, noting the difficulty of ensuring accurate surveillance.

It is difficult to adequately determine whether the successes of the ABC campaign were a result of its emphasis on changing sexual behavior, especially when one accounts for evidence that there was inconsistent application of the ABC concept. One anthropologist recounts how some churches (in Zimbabwe) that were claiming to follow the ABC model were in fact distorting its message. He describes a local church workshop for unmarried young adults where ABC was translated as A for abstinence, B for be faithful, and C for "if you cannot commit yourself to abstinence, then change—in other words, strengthen your commitment to abstinence."[42] The workshop facilitators refused to promote condoms because they worried that people who feel safe when using condoms increase their sexual activity, making them more vulnerable to infection.

Interestingly, the empirical data do confirm the fact that sexual behaviors changed in Uganda in the period of the 67 percent AIDS decrease. The average age of sexual debut went up, and the average number of sexual partners went down. The rate of marital fidelity increased, but so did the rate of condom use, especially in "high-risk encounters."[43] It is difficult to determine which of these factors was most responsible for the reversal of Uganda's epidemic. Nevertheless, the Church has touted Uganda as evidence that prevention efforts that do not focus solely on condoms are more effective, which reinforces the Church's pragmatic justification against condom use.

## OFFICIAL STATEMENTS ABOUT CONDOMS

The first detailed official statement responding to the epidemic, issued in 1987 by the US Conference of Catholic Bishops, elucidates the origins of the contemporary Catholic responses to condoms. *The Many*

*Faces of AIDS: A Gospel Response* addresses the broad range of issues initially presented by the epidemic. What the bishops say about condoms is striking, because, though they reject condoms as contrary to Catholic teaching, they also acknowledge their responsibility to permit some education about condoms because of their role as public figures. They see themselves as having two roles—one as religious leaders, the other as public figures. This distinction between their "religious" and "public" roles enables them to walk a fine line between promoting sexual abstinence as the most morally acceptable method of disease prevention and accepting a responsibility to promote condoms.

They reject the approach known as "safe sex" because they claim it "compromises human sexuality—making it safe to be promiscuous," and they argue that it is a misleading term because it is difficult to ensure that any sex will be safe. They note that "persons involved in sexual contact that is physically dangerous or morally wrong" are at the highest risk of contracting AIDS. Thus, the ultimate goal of prevention ought to be changing those behaviors through education. The bishops state that they are not interested in passing judgment on those behaviors but rather in doing what they can to protect the physical well-being of all persons. Basically, they stress that educating people about the central values of an authentic and integrated sexuality is both the most moral and the most effective way to prevent the spread of AIDS. Nevertheless, they acknowledge the difficulty of exercising their role as moral teachers in a pluralistic society, especially knowing that "some will not agree with our understanding of human sexuality." Yet they insist that AIDS prevention education ought to focus on the moral dimensions of the sexual act. In their view, this can succeed because "there are certain basic values present in our society that transcend religious or sectarian boundaries and that can constitute a common basis for these efforts."[44]

In spite of this clear position that condoms are not the solution, the bishops endorse the option of providing information about condoms, but they do so with some hesitation. They write that "educational efforts, if grounded in the broader moral vision outlined above, could include accurate information about prophylactic devices or other practices proposed by some medical experts as potential means of preventing AIDS." They further clarify this position by distinguishing the dissemination of information about condoms from the promotion of condoms. Moreover, they assert that even basic information about condoms must always be part of the broader Catholic vision of authentic human sexuality. In other words, Catholic organizations may be allowed to give people information about condoms, but they must always make clear that the only really effective way to prevent AIDS infection is "abstinence outside of marriage and fidelity within marriage." Catholic hospitals have a special responsibility to make the case for the Catholic position, but even they are permitted to inform patients that condoms are what most public officials recommend. The bishops justify this seeming contradiction by stating that though pastors ought to encourage all to live a chaste life, "if it is obvious that the person will not act without bringing harm to others, then the traditional Catholic wisdom with regard to one's responsibility to avoid inflicting greater harm may be appropriately applied."[45] In other words, they temper the concern about sexual immorality that informs the Catholic justification against condoms with concerns about harm.

Scholars have noted that in this early document the bishops appeal to the "principle of toleration"—a casuistic move that enables them to resolve this particular case (condom use for disease prevention) while also protecting the principle about condom use for contraceptive purposes.[46] Yet the principle of toleration is connected to the notion of tolerating the lesser evil—a position roundly condemned by the Vatican because it violates the principle that one may never do evil to achieve good. Toleration has been defined in this context as "a technical term related to moral agency" that "describes a situation in which a moral agent could allow one moral evil to occur with a view to avoiding a greater moral evil, while not incurring any personal responsibility for the moral evil that has been permitted."[47] In this context, the question concerns whether the good of public health can override moral concerns about condoning the use of condoms. The bishops believe that, at least in the public sphere, providing information about condoms can be tolerated. Bouchard and Pollock cite interesting theological precedents in Catholic history, such as support for the "toleration" of prostitution, Catholic just war theory, and the toleration of severe side effects from medicines that achieve a greater therapeutic good.[48]

This 1987 bishops' statement is significant because by appealing to the principle of toleration of a lesser evil, the bishops acknowledged that though the evil of contraception is a sexual sin, a condom's ability to prevent harm and potentially save a life cannot be overlooked. This attitude, however, stands as one of only a few examples of openness toward the use of condoms in the official Catholic documents. As is shown below, however, this principle, along with the principle of double effect, is the basis for strong support of condoms by many lay Catholics, Catholic theologians, and bishops' conferences. Since 1987, the

Magisterium has not supported the use of condoms or even tolerated any public education efforts that promote their use. Instead, Vatican statements have focused on attacking the efficacy of condoms and promoting abstinence education. A June 2001 statement from the Vatican to the UN General Assembly illustrates this point. The statement is intended to register the Vatican's concern about the Declaration of Commitment on HIV/AIDS adopted by the UN General Assembly. Mainly, the Vatican is concerned that the declaration overemphasizes the effectiveness of condoms in HIV/AIDS prevention. It reiterates its opposition to the use of condoms and confirms "the undeniable fact that the only safe and completely reliable method of preventing the sexual transmission of HIV is abstinence before marriage and respect and mutual fidelity within marriage."[49] Although the Vatican is endorsing Catholic marital values and principles, the main thrust of the statement is that condoms are not safe and reliable. The tolerance shown toward condoms evident in the 1987 statement thus disappears in later documents, and the focus turns to claims about both their ineffectiveness and the importance of modifying immoral behavior.

This argument is repeated throughout numerous official documents. One worth quoting at some length is the 2003 statement by the Symposium of Episcopal Conferences of Africa and Madagascar: "We want to educate appropriately and promote those changes in attitude and behaviour which value abstinence and self-control before marriage and fidelity within marriage. We want to become involved in affective and sexual education for life, to help young people and couples discover the wonder of their sexuality and their reproductive capacities. Out of such wonder and respect flow a responsible sexuality and method of managing fertility in mutual respect between the man and the woman."[50]

Although the statement focuses on a specific plan of action for the Catholic Church in Africa, it reflects the rhetoric of self-control and abstinence common to all official documents. Here, however, the bishops also suggest that a lack of sexual self-control will erode the relationship between a man and a woman, and ultimately degrade the meaning of sexuality. Later in the document, the bishops commit themselves to increasing the availability of resources needed to respond to the epidemic, without specifically mentioning condoms. The rest of the document vigorously affirms the Church's commitment to pursuing greater access to medicine and treatment for victims of the epidemic.

The question of whether the Church ought to commend the use of condoms for HIV/AIDS prevention continues to be a contentious issue well into the twenty-first century. Pope John Paul II reiterated the Church's view on the issue of condom use to prevent HIV/AIDS shortly before he died in 2005. His comments on the issue were brief and a bit opaque, yet they capture much of the persistent ambiguity about the Church's justification of its view: "The Holy See considers that in order to combat this [HIV/AIDS] disease responsibly, it is first necessary to increase its prevention, in particular by teaching respect for the sacred value of life and the correct practice of sexuality. This implies chastity and fidelity. At my request, the Church has also mobilized projects for the victims, especially to ensure that they are guaranteed access to the preventive treatment and medicines they need at numerous health care centers."[51] This passage expressed the Vatican's concern with prevention, but defined prevention narrowly as "chastity and fidelity." The reference to access to "preventive treatments" is unclear, but more recent remarks by Pope Benedict XVI make clear that the Vatican does not commend condom use as a preventive treatment.

Benedict's responses to questions about condoms drew great media attention—a fact that reinforces the importance that cultural forces exert on Church teaching. In one instance, an interviewer asked him why the Church has failed "to answer the most urgent global problems such as AIDS and overpopulation." Benedict responded by suggesting that the use of contraceptives misleads society into believing that moral problems can be solved through technical means. He distinguishes moral awareness from technical power, and he argues that both are necessary elements for advancing the development of humanity. He claims that society's problems, especially in the West, persist because moral awareness and capacity have not kept pace with advancements in technical power: "If we only teach know-how, if we only teach how to build and to use machines and how to use contraceptives, then we should not be surprised when we find ourselves facing wars and AIDS epidemics; because we need two dimensions."[52] Thus, in his view, though contraceptives might provide a technical solution, they do nothing to build up moral values in society. In fact, his comment could be interpreted as suggesting that condoms might be responsible for the continued spread of the AIDS epidemic. This suggestion was reinforced in the fall of 2009 when, as he was traveling to Africa, the pope stated that the HIV/AIDS epidemic "cannot be overcome by the distribution of condoms: on the contrary, they increase it." This remark led to a public outcry about the public health implications of these comments.[53]

In 2010, again in an interview setting, Benedict's words about condoms drew media attention, but this time because they appeared to point in a different direction. The interview, which was published in the volume *Light of the World*, was the occasion for great media speculation about whether the Catholic Church was changing its teaching on this issue. Although Benedict maintained his earlier position that condoms were not a solution to the AIDS epidemic, he said that condom use "in this or that case," motivated by "the intention of reducing the risk of infection, [can be] a first step in a movement toward a different way, a more human way, of living sexuality."[54] His claim that intention could matter was significant because it suggested that the use of a condom could not be evaluated apart from intention. If that is indeed what he meant, then it appeared to many observers that Benedict had changed Church teaching on this point. The Vatican promptly responded that this was not a change, and that the pope was simply making a statement about gay prostitutes to indicate how their use of condoms could be seen as a "first step in the direction of a moralization, a first assumption of responsibility."[55] These comments implied that the purpose of condoms for gay prostitutes was not simply to prevent infection, but that it could also be a tool toward the goal of making them more morally responsible.

The official Vatican response that no change in teaching had occurred still left many wondering whether the pope intended to loosen the strict prohibition on condoms. Benedict did not elaborate on these three interviews, and as of this writing his successor, Francis, has yet to comment specifically on the issue of the permissibility of condom use in cases of serodiscordant HIV-infected couples.[56] So as far as the official teaching of the Church on this matter, the prohibition against condoms still remains. These statements illustrate how three types of interrelated arguments are used to bolster the position. First, condoms simply fail and are thus not effective at preventing AIDS. Second, emphasizing condoms ignores the more serious issue of sexual immorality. And third, relying on condoms as the solution overlooks the deeper structural problems that have contributed to the spread of the epidemic, especially in developing countries. These three arguments coincide with the framework that I have suggested governs Catholic thought about contraception. Effectiveness correlates with concerns about harm;

sexual immorality refocuses the issue to a matter of sexual ethics; and concerns about structural problems in society correlate with social justice and the common good.

Although the arguments are not always easy to separate from one another, the first two are deployed more commonly. Yet as recently as 2009, one can see this third type of reason applied to opposition to condom distribution—here, in a non-HIV/AIDS-related context. Bishop William Murphy, chair of the US Episcopal Conference's Committee on Domestic Justice and Human Development, urged members of the US Congress to oppose a measure in President Obama's economic stimulus package that was intended to expand family planning coverage for low-income women. He writes that the Church opposes this expansion in coverage because it "neglect[s] women's real needs." His point is that the real problem for these women is not a lack of access to family planning but rather a lack of basic and essential goods needed to survive.[57]

## THE ARGUMENT AGAINST CONDOMS

We have already seen how the Church utilizes various justifications to support its opposition to artificial contraception more generally. In this chapter I focus on cases when contraceptive devices, condoms in particular, are used for noncontraceptive ends. Although the Church opposes these cases on the same grounds as its general prohibition of artificial contraception, it also relies on some justifications and arguments specific to this case. In fact, there are two distinct types of moral arguments in the official Catholic discourse about condoms. The following excerpt from a statement by the US Catholic bishops contains both types: "Sexual intercourse is appropriate and morally good only when, in the context of heterosexual marriage, it is a celebration of faithful love and is open to new life. The use of prophylactics to prevent the spread of HIV is technically unreliable."[58]

The first sentence clearly connects the immorality of contraception to the Church's overall view of the goods of sexual intercourse. For sexual intercourse to be morally good, three conditions must be met: The couple (male and female) must be married, they must remain faithful to one another, and each act of sexual intercourse must be open to new life. The third condition clearly precludes condoms because their use, whatever the intention, closes off (or at least greatly reduces) the possibility of new life. The point the bishops make in this first sentence is that condoms are inherently immoral because using them violates sexual moral norms, and these norms are violated, according to this logic, regardless of whether or not the condoms actually work to prevent disease. Put another way, the moral argument against condoms in this first sentence is not concerned with the promotion of public health but rather with the promotion of proper sexual behavior. By contrast, the second sentence asserts that condoms are technically ineffective. This is an empirical claim about disease prevention, which shifts the grounds of the argument from a moral basis to a pragmatic one. The juxtaposition of the language of technical reliability with the language of moral goodness in one brief passage shows the close relationship between these two types of justification.

The first type of argument about the objective morality of sexual acts is often based on the view that acts ought to be evaluated biologically or physically. This approach, which critics of the Church position refer to as "physicalism," describes a certain interpretation of natural law: "the a priori identification of the human moral act with the physical or biological aspect of the act."[59] Thus acts are interpreted merely on the basis of their physical structure with no attention to the intention. In the case of condoms, the Church holds that their use is wrong regardless of intention or circumstance, which means that it is the physical act of using the condom that is wrong.[60] So, whatever one's reasons for using a condom in an act of sexual intercourse, the fact that it physically obstructs conception seems to matter the most. In Catholic terms, it prevents the act from achieving its finality. Of course, proponents of condom use respond by arguing that intention has always mattered in Catholic moral theology, and that in the case of HIV/AIDS prevention, wanting to avoid conception deliberately is radically different from wanting to avoid contracting a deadly disease.

Some defenders of the Church's position frame the opposition to contraception in a different way, one that combines a focus on morality with what appear to be a set of consequentialist concerns not related to efficacy. For example, for Pope John Paul II and others, a sexual act where one or both partners use contraception is false because it turns the act into one based purely on pleasure and sensuality. The problem with the pure pursuit of sexual pleasure, according to John Paul II, is that it puts one in danger of treating the other person merely as a means to an end.[61] The conservative Catholic theologian William E. May elaborates on this point. He explains that "when spouses choose to use condoms they change the act they perform from one of true marital union (the marriage act) into a different kind of act." He supports this claim in two ways. First, following Pope John Paul II's view in the encyclical letter *Veritatis splendor*, May asserts that the moral species of an act is derived from "the proximate end of a deliberate decision." So when a couple freely chooses to use a condom (for whatever reason), their proximate end is the use of a condom while engaging in intercourse. Although they have a "further" or "more remote" end—to avoid transmitting HIV/AIDS—it is the proximate end that shapes the moral species of the act. This further end, though good, does not affect the moral species or meaning of the act.[62]

May also argues against condoms using a justification based on the "true" meaning of the sexual act. He claims that a truly authentic and moral sex act must be one where the bodies of husband and wife "speak the language of a mutual giving and receiving."[63] According to this view, the use of a condom withholds the total gift of self and thus uses the other person merely as a means to an end. Derived from John Paul II's *Theology of the Body*, the basic claim is that a sex act "deprived of its interior truth because it is artificially deprived of its procreative capacity, ceases to be an act of love."[64] In this view, the deliberate interference with "procreative capacity" deprives the sexual act of its moral meaning. We shall see this appeal to procreative capacity again in some of the early debates about the birth control pill discussed in chapter 4. This is tied to the notion of respect for the dignity of the human person understood as a unity of body and soul. This point is central in the writings of John Paul II and is also an important feature of Pope Benedict XVI's theological anthropology. Benedict writes: "Man is a being made up of body and soul. Man is truly himself when his body and soul are intimately united; the challenge of *eros* can be said to be truly overcome when this unification is achieved. Should he aspire to be pure spirit and to reject the flesh as pertaining to his animal nature alone, then spirit and body would both lose their dignity."[65]

Perhaps the most explicit connection among condoms, sexual immorality, and harm to the family is expressed in the following passage from Javier Cardinal Lozano Barragán: "Radical prevention [of AIDS] in this field must come from a correct conception and practice of sexuality, where sexual activity is understood in its deep meaning as a total and absolute expression of the fecund giving of love. This totality leads us to the exclusiveness of its exercise in marriage, which is unique and indissoluble. Secure prevention in this field thus lies in the intensification of the solidity of the family. *This is the profound meaning of the Sixth Commandment* of the law of God, which constitutes the fulcrum of the authentic prevention of AIDS in the field of sexual activity" (emphasis added).[66] Barragán is suggesting that promoters of condoms, even when motivated by the noble aim of disease prevention, are really condoning sexual promiscuity and infidelity. The Church's opposition to condoms provides it with a platform from which to promote its sexual ethic. Thus its stance is not merely a "no" to condoms but rather a "yes" to the chastity and fidelity that matter from the perspective of the Church.[67]

The second type of argument noted in the National Conference of Catholic Bishops quotation focuses on the ineffectiveness of condoms. Like the moral argument, this type of argument takes different forms—one more focused on the technical unreliability of condoms, the other more focused on whether AIDS can be controlled simply through condom use instead of through behavior modification. The first form is a claim that condoms themselves are not 100 percent reliable in stopping the spread of the virus, either because the condoms fail or because they are not used properly. The most elaborate Vatican statement on the empirical evidence against condom effectiveness was Alfonso Cardinal López Trujillo's 2003 statement "Family Values versus Safe Sex."[68] There, he presents the usual Catholic view on this issue, but he points to medical literature that raises questions about condoms' effectiveness. In particular, he notes studies that question whether the AIDS virus can infiltrate the latex in condoms. Although most public health literature has since discounted such claims about the ineffectiveness of condoms, Trujillo's main point in 2003 was that the campaigns to encourage condoms did not mention the possibility that they might fail.[69] He writes: "Given that AIDS is a serious threat, any inadequate information based on false security offered by condoms used as prophylactics would be a grave irresponsibility."[70]

The second form of the message that condoms are ineffective is premised on the belief that condom use does not change long-term behavior and will thus fail in stopping the epidemic. This form of the argument about the unreliability of condoms essentially combines a moral concern (condoms promote promiscuity) with a pragmatic concern (condom education will not stop the epidemic). As I have already noted, the Church believes that the AIDS epidemic will continue unless individuals radically alter their sexual behaviors, because, in its view, the root of the AIDS epidemic is promiscuity and infidelity. It believes that couples in monogamous relationships are less likely to be infected, and hence a more effective and long-term solution is to insist on changing sexual behaviors in regions where AIDS is rampant. As one cleric states, the Catholic Church has a "desire to identify more than technical or temporary solutions to this pandemic and, alternatively, to identify solutions based on values and on long-term behavior change on the level of relationships between individuals and in society as a whole." He says further that "regrettably, however, many scientists, HIV prevention educators, and AIDS activists are so fixed on condom promotion that they do not give due attention to the risk avoidance that is possible to achieve through abstinence outside marriage and mutual, lifelong fidelity within marriage."[71] The failure, in this second version, is not focused on the integrity or effectiveness of the condoms themselves but rather on the insidious effects of the condom promotion message, namely, that it condones sexual promiscuity. In Trujillo's words, "safe sex" campaigns are an "invitation to promiscuity."[72]

These justifications that focus on the effectiveness of condoms also follow a consequentialist type of reasoning insofar as they argue for or against the legitimacy of moral acts based on the goodness or badness of the consequences the act produces. In the official statements discussed above, for example, it is clear that there is a concern that though condoms might be useful for preventing disease, their use leads to bad consequences. This point, which Pope Paul VI mentions explicitly in *Humanae vitae*, is still present in John Paul II's and Benedict's statements.[73] They all worry that allowing persons to use artificial contraceptives will lead to hedonistic attitudes toward sex, whereby people will view others merely as a means to the end of sexual pleasure. The US Catholic bishops concurred when they rejected the concept of "safe sex" on the basis that it "compromises human sexuality—making it safe to be promiscuous."[74]

There is, however, another type of consequence that influences the Catholic response to condom use. The hierarchy is concerned about the effect that changing or revising the teaching on contraception will have on the Church's authority. In other words, if this case is deemed an exception to an objective moral principle, then the very objectivity of the principle and the Church's authority to proclaim any principle as objective are under threat. The *Humanae vitae* period of Catholic history showed us that Church leaders were truly concerned about maintaining and protecting the tradition and the objectivity of its moral norms. On one reading, contraception was not really the issue at stake with *Humanae vitae*, but rather it was Church authority.[75] To change a long-standing teaching or to allow for exceptions might erode the confidence of the faithful in the objective truth of moral norms. If the Church were to condone condom use in these cases, it might find it difficult to maintain a firm moral line. The need to maintain such a line seems most urgent for the Catholic tradition in matters of sexuality. Thus it makes sense that the Church is concerned about the possible consequences of an exception for condoms as disease prevention. The underlying point, of course, is the Church's belief that sexually transmitted diseases are caused by sexual immorality, thus any solution to the epidemic must target sexual behavior.

It will not strike many as surprising that this argument, along with the more prudential or pragmatic ones already cited, are all grounded in Catholic teaching about the objective truth of the sexual act and the connection between that truth and the purposes of marriage. Yet what is surprising is that this is not the sole, or even always the central, argument on which the Church relies. By claiming that condoms are simply not effective in stemming the tide of AIDS, the Church engages in a very different type of discourse—one that is more focused on practical public health matters. By addressing the effectiveness of condoms as part of disease prevention efforts, the Church asserts its expertise in health care delivery and public health. This raises an additional set of questions about the meaning of authority in this context. Even more significant, however, is that the Church reveals its concerns about harm and justice by using this discourse of effectiveness. This reinforces one of my central claims: that discourses about sexuality can never be separated from discourses about violence (harm) and justice.

## THEOLOGIANS DEBATE THE MAGISTERIAL POSITION

The official "magisterial" voice represents one aspect of the Catholic view. Although this voice is imbued with great authority in the Catholic tradition, other theological voices offer a different vantage point from which to understand Catholic morality. In this section I note two important trends among these voices. One attempts to conserve the Church's teaching opposing condom use; the other supports the use of condoms utilizing traditional Catholic principles. Thus both positions claim an authentic connection to the tradition while arriving at different conclusions. The aim of this analysis is to show that the difference between these two positions rests on their different views about the relationship of sex to harm and to justice.

The precise role of theologians, especially their latitude for dissent, is a contested point for many Catholics.[76] When Pope Benedict XVI was still Joseph Cardinal Ratzinger, he described the vocation of the theologian as follows: "His role is to pursue in a particular way an ever deeper understanding of the Word of God found in the inspired Scriptures and handed on by the living Tradition of the Church. He does this in communion with the Magisterium which has been charged with the responsibility of preserving the deposit of faith."[77] Although this pursuit of a "deeper understanding" may lead theologians to arrive at differing conclusions, recent popes have construed the latitude of theologians on some matters as quite narrow. For example, Richard McCormick cites John Paul II's statement that "what is taught by the Church on contraception does not belong to material freely debatable among theologians" as an example of a return to a pre–Vatican II way of thinking about magisterial authority.[78] In spite of the Magisterium's continued attempts to silence dissenting Catholic theologians, especially on matters of sexual morality, vibrant theological conversations continue to take place.[79] In the last section of this chapter I highlight a few of these conversations for the purpose of illustrating the range of appeals that ground Catholic views about condoms.

Germain Grisez's standing vis-à-vis traditional magisterial teaching is interesting to contemplate. Although his conclusions are certainly in line with the Vatican's, he relies on an unusual brand of natural law theory that diverges quite dramatically from the Thomistic account that grounds much Catholic moral theology.[80] His voice on the issue of contraception has been especially significant for a variety of reasons. He played an important role in the drafting of *Humanae vitae* and has continued to be a staunch defender of the Catholic prohibition against contraception.[81] He bases his defense on a theory of the basic goods and

natural inclinations of humans, of which procreation is one.[82] Contraception, in his words, violates the principle "that procreation is a human
good worthy of man's pursuit, and that human acts suited to achieve
this good should be done."[83]

Grisez builds his argument by defending his view that procreation is
a natural inclination and basic good against critics who claim that it is
impossible to identify such inclinations and goods with any precision.
Although he agrees that it might be difficult to determine all the goods
that should be on his list, he claims that it is easy to see procreation as
a natural inclination and thus a basic good. First, he cites the universal-
ity of the phenomenon—people everywhere beget and raise children.
Second, he claims that procreation is a good that is the object of natural
inclination because of "the fact that from a biological point of view
the work of reproduction is the fullest organic realization of the living
substance." He continues: "Reproduction is the act of maturity and full
power. It is the act which uses the best resources of the organism. It is
the act after the completion of which the life of many organisms is
finished."[84] As further evidence that procreation is a natural inclination,
he claims that even though people are able to enjoy sexual pleasure
without procreation, they nevertheless continue to reproduce. Moreover, he argues that the knowledge that human procreation is a good is
known a priori: "Prior to deliberation and so without the possibility of
choice, everyone naturally knows that procreation is a human good and
that acts fit to attain it should be performed."[85]

Although the good of procreation is an affirmative moral norm,
according to Grisez, it certainly does not translate into a requirement
to act. Not everyone is required to contribute to a particular good such
as procreation. It is for this reason that celibacy is an acceptable option.
What is unacceptable, however, is when someone acts against a good
with "direct intent." Grisez writes: "To act directly against any of the
basic human goods is to spurn one aspect of the total possibility of
human perfection, and it is freely to set the will at odds with its own
principles of interest in the goods open to us."[86] The common type of
scenario people imagine for a justified case of acting against a basic
good is in situations where two or more goods conflict. Grisez believes,
however, that an agent incurs the positive obligation to act for the good
of procreation when an individual accepts a certain role in life and then
refuses to pursue the goods appropriate to that role. For example, "the
scholar who never pursues truth, the public official who makes no effort

to improve human community, and the married couple who prefer permanent sterility to fruitfulness."[87]

Grisez presses in a slightly different direction by drawing an analogy between one's moral obligation to avoid direct contraception once one has chosen to engage in sexual intercourse and a physician's moral obligation to never directly kill a patient, even if the physician has prolonged the patient's life unnecessarily. He describes the case as follows: A physician has care of a terminal cancer patient who will die regardless of treatment. The physician, according to Grisez, has no obligation to pursue every means possible to keep the patient alive, but if he does undertake extraordinary means, he cannot "now intervene by administering an antidote in order to prevent his own previous act from continuing to have its now undesired life-giving effect." His position is based on his view that there is a clear moral line between allowing a patient to die and killing a patient. Grisez's point here is that while the death of the patient can be a hoped-for outcome, the fact that the physician has chosen to act by pursuing the extraordinary measures means that "there now no longer is an alternative he could choose consistently. He can only let the good be or set himself directly against it."[88]

Grisez then claims that though no one is obliged to have sexual intercourse, if one does choose to engage in sexual intercourse, then one has a firm obligation to act in such a way so as not to prevent procreation. To violate this obligation would, in his terms, be to act directly against a basic good. He is clear that it is perfectly acceptable to engage in sexual intercourse for "excellent reasons which have nothing to do with procreation." The point simply is that even if one's intentions are anti-procreative, *one's actions can never be*. Thus Grisez distinguishes between the person who avoids intercourse because he or she does not want to procreate from the person who actively does something to render a sexual act nonprocreative. In the former case, simply deciding to not seek a good is not the same as not loving that good. In the latter, the willed act is incompatible with loving the good of procreation.[89] It is this argument that allows Grisez and the Church to accept and promote natural family planning as a legitimate method of contraception.

It is worth noting that although Grisez addresses a married couple's use of a condom to reduce the risk of transmitting HIV, he claims that its sinfulness does not result from the fact that it is contraceptive. In fact, he claims that "using a condom is contraceptive if, and only if, the condom is used with the intention of impeding procreation."[90] The gravity of the act results from the fact that Grisez believes that sexual intercourse using a condom is not marital intercourse because it "does not pertain to procreation." In other words, sexual intercourse only counts as "good"—that is, "marital"—if it remains open to procreation. He claims that once a condom is introduced, then couples' only interest in the sexual act is to achieve orgasm. This goal is only justifiable in the context of marital intercourse (i.e., intercourse that is open to procreation). Marital intercourse, in Grisez's view, must meet four conditions: (1) It must involve a married couple; (2) it cannot be coerced; (3) it must result in ejaculation by the husband; and (4) it must be sexual intercourse, which he defines as follows: "The male's penis enters the female's vagina and is stimulated by movement and contact until the male's ejaculation occurs."[91] Thus the husband must ejaculate semen into his wife's vagina. If that fails to happen, as would be the case for a couple using a condom, then the very nature of the act is changed. Hence Grisez's response to the case of whether married couples can use condoms to protect against the spread of HIV is to move the discussion away from whether the intent is or is not contraceptive. He focuses instead on a particular biological description of what constitutes an authentic act of marital sexual intercourse. This view reinforces the kind of "physicalism" described above, but its justification is also based on a theory of natural inclinations that sees procreation as a good that can never be deliberately impeded.

Martin Rhonheimer, as a Swiss priest of Opus Dei, draws on the New Natural Law Theory associated with Grisez and others to arrive at some distinctive conclusions, especially as regards contraception.[92] Like Grisez, Rhonheimer is a traditionalist who supports the magisterial teachings opposing artificial contraception. But he believes that the matter of whether a married couple can licitly use condoms to prevent HIV infection is a complex question that "is not yet clearly settled by the Magisterium of the Church."[93] Arguing against Grisez, he holds that sexual intercourse while using a condom in the case of a married couple can certainly be called a marital act. He rejects Grisez's view because he believes it to be a "relic of an older view, focused on seeing the evil of contraception in the frustration of natural patterns, of its destroying the physical aptitude of sexual intercourse to be generative." The problem, in Rhonheimer's view, is that Grisez is drawing an implicit analogy between what he calls "condomistic sex" and sex acts that the Catholic tradition has characterized as against nature; that is, acts that utilize sexual organs in ways that are not generative, such as sodomy and masturbation. Rhonheimer claims that this analogy is counterintuitive because acts such as sodomy and masturbation are physically structured to preclude procreation, whereas the use of a condom is a human intervention. The act itself is structurally a generative act, according to Rhonheimer. Thus, one cannot assess the morality of condom use by referring to the physical act itself. Instead, one needs to determine the intentionality of the act. Rhonheimer writes: "To know what kind of human—that is, intentional—act is being performed, one must know the purpose for which this modification that physically impedes insemination has been brought about."[94]

Rhonheimer also claims that one cannot logically judge a physical device, the condom in this case, as a moral or immoral means without knowing more about the end to which it is being used. It is the nature of the "act of using" an object that determines its morality, not the physical object itself. Thus, Rhonheimer writes that it would be mistaken to consider a condom a "means" in the "moral sense," because "morally speaking a 'means' is an *action chosen to achieve a further goal*."[95] Rhonheimer's point is that determining whether the use of a condom is or is not morally licit must be based on its basic "intentionality." In other words, we must know what the intended "further goal" of a condom's use is in a particular situation.[96]

Now, to be clear, Rhonheimer is not an enthusiastic proponent of condom use in these cases. Indeed, he thinks that there are strong prudential reasons to oppose them and to advise serodiscordant couples to abstain from sex completely. Nevertheless, he rejects Grisez's argument that sex with a condom cannot be truly "marital" sex. His view, however, shows an inner tension in the Catholic argument against condoms. It points to a weakness in Grisez's (and most of the tradition's) overly biological vision of what constitutes a legitimate act of marital intercourse. It is clear that Rhonheimer, though not wanting to reduce all morality to intentionality, is concerned that Grisez's vision leaves no room to understand how intention can shape our moral acts. Though Grisez continues to frame the issue of condoms and disease prevention as a moral issue related to proper sexual behavior, Rhonheimer's argument leans toward framing it as a pragmatic issue related to what works best to prevent disease.

Grisez and Rhonheimer represent a thin slice of the spectrum of active Catholic theologians commenting on this issue. Perhaps one of the most vocal and influential theologians writing on this issue is the Jesuit James Keenan. He has played a central role in insuring that the issue of HIV/AIDS remains at the forefront of the consciousness of Catholic moral theologians, especially in North America. Along with Lisa Cahill, Margaret Farley, and others, he has taken on the issues of condom use and needle-exchange programs and has written eloquently about authentically Catholic solutions to these moral issues. In a 1999 article, Keenan lays out the historical and methodological framework that informs his approach. Following the thought of Bruno Schüller, Keenan argues that the Catholic Church experienced two distinct periods of casuistry—one in the sixteenth century, the other in the seventeenth century—which led to two very different methodological processes. According to Keenan, the sixteenth century was a time of discovery when the Church was confronted with new issues. It developed casuistry as a way to navigate through the thicket of these new cases. The navigation involved the creation of new material principles to cover the new cases. Keenan writes: "It is important for us to realize that in the 16th century, moralists and ethicists did not simply raise questions by cases; they also established standards through cases. Casuistry was not simply the art of making exceptions; it was, in fact, a method for navigating safely through the different, challenging issues on the moral horizon."[97]

This inductive mode of casuistry is valuable, according to Keenan, because of its translucence and practicality. It is translucent in the sense that "it reveals to us how we can and do agree and disagree with one another."[98] Because the focus is on cases rather than on ideologies or methodologies, persons can converge on the level of specific judgments, and this ultimately contributes to building communities. The sixteenth century was a time where this type of casuistry flourished because of the need to actually revise and create material norms and principles. The movement from cases to principles in the sixteenth century led to a different situation in the seventeenth century. Gone was the creative, imaginative casuistry described by Keenan. Instead, moralists were faced with the difficult task of simultaneously maintaining the absolute status of the law while respecting the spirit that animates it.[99] They were now engaged in a different enterprise; instead of norm building, they were applying norms to cases. The inductive thrust was inverted and replaced with a more deductive activity. This led to the development of another type of casuistry—the casuistry of accommodation—which was governed by five methodological principles: double effect, the lesser evil, cooperation in wrong-doing, totality, and toleration.

This casuistry of accommodation was designed to stretch the principles in compassionate directions without requiring the type of chaotic upheaval of established principles characteristic of the sixteenth century. In Keenan's language, the casuistry of accommodation allows for a balance between "preserving moral order and entertaining the chaos" of complex moral problems in all areas of life.[100] Keenan's point is that this history of open casuistry in Catholic moral theology reveals the willingness of the tradition to acknowledge moral chaos and to affirm that such an acknowledgment need not lead a Catholic down the path of scandal. Against this historical background, Keenan posits the claim that the official Catholic teaching has ignored this history in the face of the moral chaos wrought by HIV/AIDS. It has ignored it by resisting and condemning Catholic theologians engaged in this "traditional" casuistry to sort through the moral dimensions of the HIV/AIDS epidemic. Keenan's astonishment at the Church's resistance is compounded by the fact that he claims that these theologians (himself included) are utilizing the tamer seventeenth-century version of casuistry. He writes: "The church leadership is not currently resisting foundational challenges; rather, it is resisting the casuistry of accommodation that so significantly helped build up the Catholic community over the past 400 years."[101]

Regarding the case of condom distribution, Keenan reviews the US Conference of Catholic Bishops' statement *The Many Faces of AIDS* and concludes that the bishops utilize the principle of toleration in the section of the document described earlier in this chapter as controversial.[102] He notes that they had used such an accommodating principle when they crafted their position on nuclear deterrence. Thus, in a similar way, the bishops could protect a material principle (concerning illicit sex) while resolving a new case. As I pointed out above, the bishops pulled back from this position in later statements. Keenan believes that the church's response to this case, along with the case of needle exchange as HIV/AIDS prevention, is illuminated by another Catholic position about AIDS: the institution by many US male religious orders of required HIV testing as part of the application. Keenan argues that the bishops' resistance to accommodate AIDS prevention and testing betrays a deeper anxiety about the disease and the specific effects it might have on the Catholic Church—basically an attitude of self-protection. In Keenan's view, the bishops are concerned with the infection of the Church body both literally and figuratively. Their literal concerns are characterized by the mandated testing for all seminary applicants and their figurative concerns by the resistance against condoms. Keenan writes about the bishops: "They were concerned with whether preventive measures against the infection could in turn infect traditional principles on marriage, sex, and drug use."[103]

Lisa Cahill also supports the use of condoms for prevention in the context of HIV/AIDS by relying on traditional Catholic principles. She claims that AIDS is not a sexual issue, and hence is not only about sexual autonomy but also an issue of poverty and sexism, which are both issues of justice.[104] She also relies on a traditional Catholic argument based on the rule of double effect to argue that contraception is not a directly intended effect of the act, but rather a "side effect." In her view, the avoidance of AIDS ought to be construed as the directly intended effect. One can then apply the principle of proportionality (traditionally the fourth element of double effect) to argue that the human life saved is a proportionate good.[105] Of course, the problem with this line of reasoning is that it overlooks the fact that the Vatican views contraception as an intrinsically evil act, and thus it can never be an intended or even a merely foreseen effect of the act. The Vatican's view about the intrinsic evil of contraception is partly grounded in the belief that using a condom while engaged in sex changes the nature of the act. The use of contraceptives with the intent to prevent conception is thus intrinsically evil. Yet, it is important to note an inconsistency here in the Vatican position. The use of condoms in the context of HIV/AIDS prevention is not intended to prevent pregnancy. In other words, there is no anti-procreative intent. This is a case of the use of a contraceptive device (a condom) for therapeutic purposes. One way to frame the inconsistency is to view it as an example of overlapping justifications; yet this does not address important questions about the role of intention in evaluations of contraception. Keenan and Cahill appeal to traditional Catholic principles such as cooperation and double effect. They also conform to the Catholic norms of justice and the common good by viewing HIV/AIDS as primarily an issue of justice rather than an issue of sex. Cahill writes: "AIDS as a justice issue concerns the social relationships that help spread HIV and fail to alleviate AIDS, relationships of power and vulnerability that are in violation of Catholic norms of justice and the common good."[106]

This brief sampling of recent theological voices on the issue of whether condom use can ever be licit points to a key question for interpreting Catholic discourses on contraception. Is contraception immoral because it is a sexual sin, or is it immoral because it violates a recognized norm of justice? Keenan's observations help us frame the question a little differently. Does justice require accommodation? Is the inductive casuistry of norm building the just method for responding to HIV/AIDS? Cahill's identification of AIDS as a justice issue further reinforces the fact that the Magisterium's attempt to tie the use of condoms to sexual promiscuity might miss some of the richness of the tradition's own set of overlapping justifications.

## NOTES

1. Paul VI, *Humanae vitae*, par. 14.

2. The one exception is paragraph 15, which states that "the Church, on the contrary, does not at all consider illicit the use of those therapeutic means truly necessary to cure diseases of the organism, even if an impediment to procreation, which may be foreseen, should result therefrom, provided such impediment is not, for whatever motive, directly willed." Here the issue concerns disease treatment. *Humanae vitae*, par.15.

3. Ibid., par. 11.

4. The Catholic Church prohibits artificial contraception in all cases because of its belief that engaging in a sexual act while using a contraceptive is objectively wrong and therefore always an evil. In other words, no circumstance or motive alters the fact that the object of the will—to engage in an act that intentionally (knowingly) impedes the possibility of new life—is evil. The *Catechism* quotes the following passage from the Vatican II document *Gaudium et spes*: "The morality of the behavior does not depend on sincere intention and evaluation of motives alone; but it must be determined by objective criteria, criteria drawn from the nature of the person and his acts, criteria that respect the total meaning of mutual self-giving and human procreation in the context of true love"; *Catechism*, par. 2368.

5. See the discussion of such a case given by Keenan, "Applying the Seventeenth-Century Casuistry of Accommodation to HIV Prevention," 492.

6. A serodiscordant couple is one wherein one partner has tested positive for HIV and the other has not.

7. By "unofficial discussions," I mean articles and statements issued by theologians and lay Catholics who are not writing as representatives of the Magisterium.

8. This group edited a highly influential volume of essays; see Cahill et al., *Catholic Ethicists on HIV/AIDS Prevention.*

9. Fuller and Keenan, "Introduction," 29.

10. Marchetto, *HIV/AIDS and Its Effects.*

11. Fuller and Keenan, "Introduction," 29.

12. For a good overview of many aspects of the early history, see McKenzie, *AIDS Reader.*

13. This information is from Avert, "Worldwide HIV & AIDS Statistics," www.avert.org/worldstats.htm.

14. According to the Centers for Disease Control and Prevention, "In 2009, African Americans comprised 14% of the US population but accounted for 44% of all new HIV infections and Latinos accounted for 20% of new HIV infections in the United States while representing approximately 16% of the total US population"; www.cdc.gov/hiv/topics/aa/index.htm and www.cdc.gov/hiv/latinos/index .htm.

15. This information is from World Health Organization, "Global Summary of the AIDS Epidemic 2011," www.who.int/hiv/data/2012_epi_core_en.png.

16. Although the evidence does show that the disease may have begun in Africa, much of the early attention in the 1980s was on North American populations.

17. Sub-Saharan Africa is the most affected region, with nearly one in every twenty adults living with HIV. Sixty-nine percent of all people living with HIV are living in this region; these data are from www.who.int/mediacentre/factsheets/ fs360/en/index.html.

18. In early 2013, scientists announced at a professional meeting that an infant infected with the HIV virus that causes AIDS had been successfully cured. At this point, the findings have yet to be published in a peer-reviewed scientific journal. This fueled speculation that a cure for the disease might be an achievable goal. See Pollack and McNeil, "In Medical First, a Baby with HIV Is Deemed Cured."

19. For more information on the benefits of antiretroviral therapy, see Centers for Disease Control and Prevention, "Prevention Benefits of HIV Treatment," www.cdc.gov/hiv/topics/treatment/resources/factsheets/tap.htm.

20. Kelly, "AIDS and Ethics."

21. Ibid., 332.

22. Zuger, "AIDS on the Wards," 18.

23. Kelly's discussion of this issue really dates his article; see Kelly, "AIDS and Ethics," 334–35.

24. See, e.g., Cohen-Kohler, "Morally Uncomfortable Global Drug Gap."

25. Kowalewski, "Religious Constructions," 91.

26. Men who have sex with men are still the largest risk group for contracting the disease. Statistics from the Centers for Disease Control and Prevention show that in 2009 (the most recent year with full data), 61 percent of those infected with HIV were men who had sex with men. See Centers for Disease Control and Prevention, "Gay, Bisexual, and Other Men Who Have Sex with Men," www.cdc .gov/hiv/topics/msm.

27. Vitillo, *Action in Response.*

28. Barragán, "Message on the Occasion of World AIDS Day."

29. Riedemann, "African View of Church and HIV."

30. Caritas, "Catholic Church Serving People with HIV and AIDS," www
.caritas.org/activities/hiv_aids/the_catholic_church_serving_people_with_hiv_and
_aids.html.

31. CELAM Office of Justice and Solidarity, "Pastoral Strategy."

32. This was according to the US Food and Drug Administration in 1990.

33. UNAIDS.

34. Swanson, "Beyond Condoms."

35. Riedemann, "African View of Church and HIV."

36. Meassick, "HIV/AIDS Prevention," 184.

37. Lepani, "Fitting Condoms on Culture," 246–47.

38. Ibid.

39. For a discussion of this point, see Lepani, "Fitting Condoms on Culture."

40. Sinding, "Does 'CNN' Work Better than 'ABC'?," 38.

41. Slutkin et al., "How Uganda Reversed Its HIV Epidemic."

42. Rodlach, *Witches, Westerners, and HIV.*

43. Schoepf, "Uganda."

44. US Conference of Catholic Bishops, *Many Faces of AIDS.*

45. Ibid.

46. Fuller and Keenan, "Introduction," 23.

47. Bouchard and Pollock, "Condoms," 100.

48. Ibid., 101–2.

49. Vatican, "Statement of Interpretation."

50. Symposium of Episcopal Conferences of Africa and Madagascar, "Church
in Africa."

51. John Paul II, "Address to HE Ms. Monique Patricia Antoinette Frank."

52. Benedict XVI, "Interview of the Holy Father."

53. *The Lancet* accused the pope of "publicly distorting scientific evidence to
promote Catholic doctrine," and demanded a public retraction from the pope, writing: "When any influential person, be it a religious or political leader, makes a false
scientific statement that could be devastating to the health of millions of people,
they should retract or correct the public record." "Redemption for the Pope?" *The
Lancet*, 2009, 373:1054.

54. Benedict XVI, *Light of the World*, 119.

55. Ibid.

56. In an interview conducted in August 2013, Pope Francis said the following
about the Catholic Church's view on contraception: "We cannot insist only on
issues related to abortion, gay marriage, and the use of contraceptive methods. This
is not possible. I have not spoken much about these things, and I was reprimanded
for that. But when we speak about these issues, we have to talk about them in a
context. The teaching of the Church, for that matter, is clear, and I am a son of
the Church, but it is not necessary to talk about these issues all the time." Spadaro,

"Big Heart Open to God," 26. Some interpreted these remarks as an indication that Pope Francis is open to change. However, there is nothing in the interview that suggests an explicit direct change in the Catholic teaching about contraception.

57. US Conference of Catholic Bishops, "Bishops Urge Congress to Make the Poor a Priority."

58. National Conference of Catholic Bishops, *Called to Compassion*, pt. IV, sec. 3.

59. Curran, *Catholic Moral Theology*, 104.

60. Pope John Paul II defended the Church from the charge of "physicalism." In *Veritatis splendor*, he wrote: "A doctrine which dissociates the moral act from the bodily dimensions of its exercise is contrary to the teaching of Scripture and Tradition" (par. 49). He also states, "Therefore this law [natural law] cannot be thought of as simply a set of norms on the biological level; rather it must be defined as the rational order whereby man is called by the Creator to direct and regulate his life and actions and in particular to make use of his own body" (par. 50).

61. Karol Wojtyla (Pope John Paul II) wrote: "If the possibility of parenthood is deliberately excluded from marital relationship, the character of the relationship between the partners automatically changes. The change is away from unification in love and in the direction of mutual, or rather, bilateral, 'enjoyment.'" Also: "Willing acceptance of the possibility of procreation in the marital relationship safeguards love and is an indispensable condition of a truly personal union." Wojtyla, *Love and Responsibility*, 228, 230.

62. May, "Catholic Health Care," 1–2.

63. Ibid.

64. John Paul II, *Theology of the Body*, 398.

65. Benedict XVI, *Deus caritas est*, par. 5.

66. Barragán, "Message on the Occasion of World AIDS Day."

67. To clarify the logic, the following analogy might be useful. Today, persons with high cholesterol levels are routinely prescribed statin drugs that are intended to reduce levels of cholesterol in the blood. In most cases physicians also suggest exercise and diet, and other lifestyle changes. Thus, whereas conventional medical wisdom recognizes that changing behaviors is ultimately the most effective treatment, it does not prohibit the use of "artificial means" of reducing cholesterol levels. Though this is not an exact analogy, it captures the point about whether allowing for condoms as disease prevention actually promotes promiscuous sexual behaviors.

68. Trujillo, "Family Values."

69. See, e.g., Warner et al., "Condom Use."

70. Trujillo, "Family Values," par. 6.

71. Swanson, "Beyond Condoms."

72. Trujillo, "Family Values,"

73. Paul VI, *Humanae vitae*, par. 17.

74. National Conference of Catholic Bishops, *Called to Compassion*, sec. IV, par. 3.

75. See Kalbian, "Catholics and Contraception."

76. For an excellent discussion of teaching authority, see Sullivan, *Magisterium*, esp. chap. 8.

77. Ratzinger, *Instruction*, par. 6.

78. McCormick, *Critical Calling*, 162.

79. For a recent example of magisterial control over theological discourse on sexual ethics, see "Notification of the Congregation for the Doctrine of the Faith."

80. Salzman and Lawler, *Sexual Person*, 48–92.

81. Grisez has written extensively on this topic. See Grisez, *Contraception*.

82. Grisez lists the following as basic goods: life, knowledge, holiness or religion, self-integration, justice, friendship, and skill in work or play that enriches human life.

83. Grisez, *Contraception*, 76.

84. Ibid., 79.

85. Ibid., 80.

86. Ibid., 83.

87. Ibid., 86.

88. Ibid., 89–90.

89. Ibid., 91.

90. Grisez, "Moral Questions," 471.

91. Ibid., 472.

92. For a good overview of Rhonheimer's sexual ethics, see Salzman and Lawler, *Sexual Person*.

93. Guevin and Rhonheimer, "On the Use of Condoms," 40.

94. Ibid., 44.

95. Ibid., 45.

96. Rhonheimer distinguishes various senses of intention. His concern is with the category of *praeter intentionem*, defined as what is "beside," "outside," or "beyond" intention. He thinks that *Humanae vitae*'s allowance for the use of anovulants for therapeutic purposes is a useful analogy to the condoms as disease prevention case. See my discussion in chapter 4 of the present volume. Rhonheimer, 41.

97. Keenan, "Applying the Seventeenth-Century Casuistry of Accommodation to HIV Prevention," 494.

98. Ibid., 495.

99. Ibid., 497.

100. Ibid., 500.

101. Ibid., 501.

102. See US Conference of Catholic Bishops, *Many Faces of AIDS*.

103. Keenan, "Prophylactics."

104. Cahill, "AIDS, Justice, and the Common Good," 282.

105. Cahill, *Theological Bioethics*, 158–59.

106. Cahill, "AIDS, Justice and the Common Good," 282.

# CHAPTER 4

# VIOLENCE
## Emergency Contraception
## and Rape

I T MAY COME AS A SURPRISE that the Catholic Church in the United States allows its hospitals to dispense emergency contraceptives for rape victims. Is this position at odds with the Church's absolute prohibition of artificial contraception? As we have seen in this study, the magisterial teaching asserts that it is the *physical* act of using artificial contraception to directly impede procreation that is intrinsically evil. In other words, it is not merely a matter of whether one intends to prevent a sexual act from achieving its procreative finality. In the language of Catholic moral theology, this means that the act of engaging in sexual intercourse while using a contraceptive is objectively wrong, regardless of one's intentions or the circumstances of the particular situation; it is an intrinsically evil act.[1] We have seen how this type of position leads the Church to assert that the use of condoms, even by married people who want to prevent each other from being infected by HIV, is morally wrong. Moreover, we saw that it is primarily the discourse of sexual immorality that frames the Church's view on that issue. Thus, instead of focusing on how condoms might reduce harm or distribute harms more justly, the Church worries mainly about how condoms might lead to more promiscuous sexual behavior. In this chapter we turn to a case that highlights violence and the just distribution of harms as the central issues at stake in contraception.

The answer to the question of why the Church allows for the use of emergency contraception for rape victims lies in a long history of Catholic interpretations of a set of related issues: rape, resistance to rape, therapeutic uses of birth control, and problematic cases related to contraception. Put briefly, however, the Church concludes that the act of preventing the aggressor's sperm from fertilizing the victim's egg does not count as an act of contraception because rape is not truly an act of sexual intercourse; thus a woman can legitimately "defend" herself from the unjust aggression of the rapist's sperm. However, the Church holds that if the sperm has already fertilized an egg, then any attempt to destroy the embryo is illicit. Thus the Church allows for emergency contraceptives in this case, as long as there is no possibility of harm to an embryo. Yet most of the rhetoric about emergency contraception claims that it results in the destruction of embryos. This poses a serious contradiction. Although there is a clear distinction between preventing fertilization and destroying an embryo, the Church has argued in such a way as to deny that distinction. In other words, it claims that emergency contraception deliberately destroys embryos, except when discussing the case of its use in rape. For the most part, the Church remains unconvinced by the medical evidence that overwhelmingly confirms that these interventions work as contraceptives to prevent an egg from being fertilized by a sperm. Yet by supporting the use of emergency contraceptives for rape victims, they are acknowledging that emergency contraception does prevent the sperm from fertilizing the egg rather than destroying the embryo.

Put more simply, if the Church asserts that all emergency contraceptives cause abortions, how can the US Catholic bishops approve their use for victims of rape? What are the implications of such a position for the Church's overall teaching on contraception? What I argue in this chapter is that this case provides one illustration of how violence functions as a central category in Catholic evaluations of contraception. Violence functions in three ways in this particular case. First, official Catholic teachings reject emergency contraceptives—mainly the morning-after pill—because of a persistent belief that they prevent pregnancies by destroying embryos; that is, they cause abortions. Second, the rape exception involves another facet of violence—not just against the embryo but also against the unjust aggressor's sperm. Third, and finally, the exception for rape rests on the interpretation that rape is violence rather than a sexual act. This enables the Church to view emergency contraceptives in this case as not really contraceptives. This chapter positions the debate about emergency contraception in two contexts: the broader cultural and scientific history of modern emergency contraception (especially the Church's consistent worry about the abortive effects of this intervention), and the rape exception and its history in the Catholic tradition. Each of these contexts adds texture to our understanding of the Church's response to this contemporary issue.

## THE DEVELOPMENT OF
## EMERGENCY CONTRACEPTION

At present in the United States, three emergency contraceptives are available to women who have unprotected sex and wish to avoid a possible pregnancy: levonorgestrel, marketed as Plan B One-Step and Next Choice; ulopristal acetate, marketed as Ella; and the Copper T3 intra-uterine device, which is marketed as Paragard.[2] Unlike traditional contraceptives, which are taken or used *prior to* sexual intercourse, these act to prevent pregnancy *after* unprotected sex or when contraceptives fail. There is a small window of time for using these treatments, usually within 120 hours after sexual intercourse. In most Western countries, including the United States, they are legal and widely available. In 2006, the US Food and Drug Administration (FDA) approved the over-the-counter sale of the emergency contraceptive Plan B to women over the age of eighteen years. By 2009, the age had been lowered to include girls under seventeen. However, there continues to be a controversy about whether young girls ought to have access without a prescription.[3]

In the mid-1960s, several years after the birth control pill was approved by the FDA and marketed in the United States, some researchers began exploring whether it could also be used immediately after sexual intercourse to prevent conception.[4] The researchers hypothesized that the pill taken in large doses would cause an initial increase in the growth of the endometrial lining, which would be sloughed off as soon as the body returned to its normal levels of estrogen. If an embryo had already been implanted, it would be destroyed and a pregnancy would be prevented. Note that this process would, according to Catholic teaching, constitute an abortion. This approach of using a large dose of the birth control pill after intercourse was the earliest phase in the development of emergency contraception. The regimen involved taking a total of four birth control pills—two within 72 hours of sex, followed by two more 12 hours later.[5] This was problematic for several reasons, including the fact that the FDA had only approved the pill for use before sex and in more limited and regulated doses.[6] Thus few doctors felt comfortable prescribing this large dose as a mode of emergency contraception. They were also concerned about the safety of this regimen, especially in light of the fact that the already high-dose pill was suspected of having serious side effects.[7]

By the 1970s, pharmaceutical companies had turned their efforts to developing and marketing a lower-dose birth control pill.[8] Although this effort was a positive one motivated by a desire to increase the safety of the pill, a lower-dose pill (even if taken in larger quantities) was less likely to work as an emergency contraceptive. As Coeytaux and Pills-bury argue, the "priorities of the pharmaceutical companies vis-à-vis 'the pill' were to put improved low-dose pills on the market—which they did. Their attention was not on after-sex emergency use of the pill."[9] Thus one consequence of the development of the lower-dose birth control pill was that scientists were forced to look for alternatives other than high doses of the birth control pill to use as emergency contraception. This resulted in the development of levonorgestrel, a progestin that relied on a different mechanism than the estrogen-based birth control pill. The idea of a progestin-only pill taken after each act of intercourse had first been discussed in the early 1970s. These early discussions were not focused on progestin's "emergency" usage; rather, researchers were interested in the possibility that this newly developed pill might replace existing birth control pills as a primary mode of birth control. The earliest findings about the effectiveness of progestins as a primary contraceptive were not encouraging, however. Thus the first FDA-approved emergency contraceptive was a combination protocol known as the "Yuzpe regime," which combined the birth control pill (estrogen/estradiol) with levonorgestrel.[10] Over time, however, research showed that levonorgestrel used alone (in either one or two doses) was just as effective, and perhaps even more effective, than the Yuzpe regime, and with fewer side effects.

It was not until the late 1990s that a much stronger progestin-only pill—Plan B—was marketed and approved by the FDA for use as a dedicated emergency contraceptive.[11] In 1999, the FDA approved Plan

B for prescription use; and in 2006, it was approved for behind-the-counter sale to women eighteen years and older. The FDA was poised to remove the age restriction, but in a charged and controversial political move, it was blocked from doing so by the health and human services secretary Kathleen Sibelius in 2011.[12] Plan B has become the most widely used emergency contraception, much preferable to other alternatives that require taking higher doses of progestin.[13] It is also the active ingredient in Norplant and Jadele, the long-acting contraceptive implants that drew a great deal of attention in the 1990s.[14]

The Catholic Church's disapproval of all these emergency contraceptive options rests primarily on concerns about their potential to destroy an embryo. As a result, much of the Catholic discourse about these pharmaceutical interventions has focused on determining what they do. Exactly how do they prevent a pregnancy? Do they merely act to block fertilization of an egg, or do they actually prevent an already fertilized egg from being implanted? The medical and scientific establishment has gained confidence that these hormonal interventions do not cause abortions. This view is supported by several studies in the past decade that demonstrate that when taken alone, Plan B does not act to prevent implantation. In fact, in one study, women who took the pill after ovulation when fertilization was most likely to occur did get pregnant. The fact that levonorgestrel was not effective in preventing implantation has lessened the concerns that many initially had about this class of drugs.[15] A recent review of scientific studies of the mechanisms of emergency contraception definitively states that "a single dose of 1.5 mg LNG [Plan B] or 30 mg UPA [Ella] acts through inhibition of or postponing ovulation but does not prevent fertilization or implantation and has no adverse effect on pregnancy."[16] Yet the Catholic Church continues to view these pills with suspicion. This suspicion is deepened by the fact that proponents of emergency contraception do not view the destruction of a pre-implantation embryo as morally problematic; in their view, it is not abortion. One medical opinion states, "Levonorgestrel does not cause abortion; it does not terminate an established pregnancy (an implanted conceptus) and should not be confused with the abortifacient mifepristone (RU-486)."[17] This statement does not mention whether the levonorgestrel prevents an already-fertilized egg from being implanted, a point that matters greatly to Catholic moralists.

The intrauterine device (IUD) and mifepristone (RU486, known as the abortion pill) are also often described in the medical literature as emergency contraceptives.[18] Both these mechanisms are more likely to have an abortifacient effect. In the case of RU486, this is precisely the effect it is intended to have, whereas the copper IUD's effect seems less certain. Earlier studies had theorized that the IUD prevents implantation of an embryo, but more recent research appears to show "that the contraceptive effect is not related to implantation, but rather to fertilization."[19] Nevertheless, the perception that IUDs destroy embryos persists in the Catholic literature. As noted above, this is due to the Catholic concern for the pre-implanted embryo—an issue that the scientific literature responds to differently than the Church does. So, for example, a 1996 study described the copper IUD as follows: "The copper IUD can also function to prevent implantation by causing an inflammatory response to the endometrium. The IUD does not act as an abortifacient and does not disrupt an already implanted embryo."[20] Again, as in the earlier statement, these authors define abortion narrowly as the destruction of an already-implanted embryo. In their view, preventing implantation is not akin to abortion, whereas the Catholic view holds that even the pre-implantation embryo ought to be protected.

A related controversy surrounding emergency contraceptives is whether or not they are effective. For the past decade the medical consensus has been that emergency contraception can be as effective as 95 percent (if taken within 24 hours of sexual intercourse) or 58 percent (if taken within 49 to 72 hours of sexual intercourse). It also appears that the success rates for the newer drugs (ulipristal acetate) might be even higher. These rates of effectiveness are, however, very difficult to measure. They are essentially estimates "based on comparing the actual number of pregnancies occurring in a cohort of women using a method of emergency contraception with the number that might have been expected without EC [emergency contraception] use."[21] Compounding the difficulties of estimating effectiveness is that women who use these contraceptives do so at various times in their cycles.[22] Both the mechanism and the effectiveness of emergency contraceptives are highly dependent on when they are used during a woman's menstrual cycle. Consequently, it is difficult to come up with a pill whose mechanism is the same in all cases. The various possible effects of these pills (to prevent ovulation, prevent fertilization, or prevent implantation) all depend on the woman's cycle. Essentially, if its function is to interfere with or block ovulation, it can only be effective if the woman is ovulating. If its function, however, is to prevent fertilization, it may be too late for a woman who is ovulating. The sperm could have reached the area of fertilization within minutes of intercourse and because treatment is usually not begun until several hours after intercourse, it is likely that a pregnancy could still occur.

## THE OFFICIAL CATHOLIC TEACHING ON EMERGENCY CONTRACEPTION

The contemporary Catholic discussion about the ethics of emergency contraception is clearly focused on the perceived scientific uncertainty regarding exactly how emergency contraceptives work. The Vatican has issued relatively few statements about the ethics of emergency contraception. The statements it has made reiterate the Catholic opposition to artificial contraception but focus more on the evil of emergency contraception as connected to abortion—that is, to its potential to harm life.

The Pontifical Academy for Life issued the first complete and definitive Vatican statement on this issue in 2000 in response to the availability of emergency contraception in Italian pharmacies. The statement's view is shaped almost entirely by the idea that emergency contraception is an abortifacient, and thus immoral. The statement characterizes the morning-after pill as "a hormone-based preparation (it contains oestrogens, oestrogen/progestogens, or only progestogens) which, within and no later than 72 hours after a presumably fertile act of sexual intercourse, has a predominantly 'anti-implantation' function."[23] It describes this function as "nothing other than a chemically induced abortion," and thus as absolutely unlawful. The statement rejects calling these drugs emergency contraceptives and chooses instead to refer to them as "the morning-after pill." This decision about terminology is meant to reinforce their view that this is not a contraceptive but rather an abortifacient. This view conforms with the Catholic belief that abortion is not limited simply to the destruction of an already-implanted embryo; it also includes the deliberate destruction of a fertilized ovum from the moment of conception, even if that ovum has yet to be implanted in the woman's uterus.[24] It is noteworthy that this statement does not mention the use of these drugs in cases of rape. The final sentence of the statement summarizes what the Vatican believes to be at stake for those who approve of these drugs. The authors describe "these procedures" as "new *hidden* forms of aggression against the weakest and most defenceless individuals, as is the case with a human embryo."[25]

The view that these contraceptives cause abortions persists in Catholic discourse. Even a more recent statement issued by the Pontifical Academy for Life in 2007 describes emergency contraception as abortive, while failing to mention the scientific debates surrounding its mechanism. The authors assert that "the effects of this form of contraception are abortive (preventing implantation or gestation)."[26] This was reiterated by the Congregation for the Doctrine of Faith in its 2008 instruction on bioethics *Dignitas personae*.[27] The authors describe emergency contraceptives as "new forms of interception and contragestation," and they assert that both these methods are, technically, methods of abortion. Methods of interception are those that "interfere with the embryo before implantation"; and countergestative methods "cause the elimination of the embryo once implanted."[28] The Instruction ignores methods that work before fertilization. It proclaims with certainty that the possibility of harm to the embryo is always present. This brief look at Vatican statements about emergency contraception shows that its view on this issue is consistent insofar as it treats the subject as a type of abortion rather than contraception, a point that is complicated by the US bishops' approval of the use of emergency contraception after rape.

One might wonder, despite mounting scientific evidence that emergency contraception does not harm embryos, why most official Catholic responses to emergency contraceptives continue to view them as abortifacients. One reason might be that the research about the mechanism of action of emergency contraception was only in its infancy in the early years of the drug's availability. The lack of studies led to uncertainty, which has made the association of emergency contraceptives with abortion a difficult one to shake. Another explanation for the Church's insistence on this as an issue related more to abortion than contraception concerns the timing of the treatment. Other methods of artificial birth control interfere with or disrupt the act of sexual intercourse. Plan B's effect, by contrast, is to disrupt the process after sexual intercourse—a period when it is difficult to determine with any certainty whether the egg has been fertilized. Finally, it also might be the case that abortion is a much more compelling and convincing issue than contraception. In other words, it is easier to convince people that destroying embryos is wrong, since for many, the act of abortion is more morally serious than an act of contraception. Thus, by continuing to stress the connection between emergency contraception and abortion, the Church is able to make a stronger case. This possibility is reinforced by the historical precedent of connecting contraception to abortion.

In fact, as I noted in chapter 2, many of the very earliest Christian condemnations of contraception drew on this fact. John Noonan's historical research shows how the early Christian sources often blurred the distinction between preventing conception and harming an already-conceived embryo. The connection was so great that some of the earliest Christian condemnations referred to contraception as a form of homicide or parricide. Although this confusion may have resulted from an inadequate grasp of the biology of reproduction, Noonan finds it more likely that it served as a rhetorical device to solidify the Christian critique of the general Roman disregard for new life. Blurring the lines between abortifacients and contraceptives served to strengthen the Christian case against both practices.[29]

It might seem that a resolution to this moral problem is impossible until the Church is convinced by the scientific evidence. Yet the persistent association of contraception and abortion in Catholic moral theology is so strong that one can imagine that even scientific certainty will not completely remove the concerns about emergency contraception. Daniel Sulmasy makes the relevant observation that a significant proportion of the science on this issue is affected by "advocate science"— the pursuit of a study to support a particular political or social agenda.[30] It is certainly possible that such agendas could fuel research on this area. It is noteworthy that in the relatively brief history of emergency contraception research, one of the main players has been the World Health Organization.[31] Its motivation is to provide easy, safe, and accessible contraception to women worldwide. Sulmasy, however, is not so concerned that the advocacy of emergency contraception is affecting the science. Rather, he notes an important principle in pharmacology; that is, that most drugs do more than one thing. This principle leads him to conclude that although the primary mechanism of emergency contraception drugs such as levonorgestrel is not abortifacient, a "residual scientific uncertainty" is likely to remain.[32]

## *The Exception in Cases of Rape*

Directive 36 of the US Catholic bishops' directives to Catholic health care institutions stands out as a possible anomaly. It clearly distinguishes the contraceptive from the abortive effects of emergency contraceptives, and thus accepts the possibility that their effect might possibly not be abortive. Writing about the context of sexual assault, the bishops state:

> Compassionate and understanding care should be given to a person who is the victim of sexual assault. Health care providers should cooperate with law enforcement officials and offer the person psychological and spiritual support as well as accurate medical information. A female who has been raped should be able to defend herself against a potential conception from the sexual assault. If, after appropriate testing, there is no evidence that conception has occurred already, she may be treated with medications that would prevent ovulation, sperm capacitation, or fertilization. It is not permissible, however, to initiate or to recommend treatments that have as their purpose or direct effect the removal, destruction, or interference with the implantation of a fertilized ovum.[33]

Two factors precipitated this statement: the increased and easy availability of Plan B and other emergency contraceptives, and the passage of legislation in numerous states requiring emergency rooms to dispense the drug or information about the drug to victims of rape. This placed pressure on Catholic hospitals to provide this treatment, especially for victims of sexual violence. In fact, as of February 2013, sixteen states and the District of Columbia have passed legislation that require hospitals to offer emergency contraception and/or provide information about it to women who have been sexually assaulted.[34]

Based on the established Catholic teaching on contraception, one would expect the Church and its health care system to oppose these pills without exception; they are, after all, contraceptives. Yet as we saw in the previous passage, this is not the case. They are permitted on two conditions: (1) The recipient of the pill must be a victim of rape, and (2) there must be certainty that she is not already pregnant. The first condition—the requirement that these pills are only licit in cases of rape—poses an interesting challenge to the Catholic view about artificial contraception. To defend this view, some moralists have turned to the history of moral theology and have noted that in the past the "expulsion of the semen" had been allowed in rape cases. The majority position historically has held that it is in fact justifiable for women to protect themselves from a pregnancy in cases of rape, on the condition that they can do so without destroying an embryo or fetus.

Notably, this right to "protection" from pregnancy does not apply to women who have not been raped. Thus, a woman's status as a rape victim sanctions her ability to interfere with the natural purposes and ends of sexual intercourse. The traditional argument about rape and contraception is built on the notion that attempting to expel or incapacitate the "seed" of the rapist is an extension of defending oneself against an unjust aggressor. Hamel and Panicola describe the traditional exception as follows: "Measures taken to prevent conception in such cases fall outside the general prohibition against contraception because the assailant's act is a violation of justice, and any semen within the woman's body is considered a continuation of the unjust aggression against which she may licitly defend herself."[35] More recently, in their ruling in favor of the use of emergency contraception for rape victims, the Catholic bishops of England and Wales asserted that taking the morning-after pill is not an act of contraception because it is an act "undertaken . . . to remove or neutralize the assailant's sperm or seminal fluid."[36] Notice that by referring to contraception simply as a response to sperm, the Church avoids any worries about the purposes and meanings of sexual acts.

The use of contraception in such cases is justified as self-defense, which presumes a strong contrast between an act of violence (rape) and a natural sexual act (marital intercourse).[37] Hence, contraception in the context of rape is a different type of act because the goods of the marriage relationship are not destroyed.[38] Essentially, because the act of rape has nothing (usually) to do with marriage, it is not deemed to be a sexual act. Unlike in the case of condoms for disease prevention, the woman's life is not at stake in this case; but rather what is at stake is the possibility of the continued injustice brought upon her by the rapist. There is no doubt in this case that the intention is contraceptive; but in essence, the Church argues that because this case is not about sex, the traditional argument no longer applies; violence becomes the governing framework for assessing this situation.

The second condition addresses the worry that these contraceptives may destroy an embryo, which, as we have noted, is a form of abortion according to Catholic teaching. This poses some practical issues for

Catholic hospitals: how to determine without a doubt whether or not an egg has been fertilized, especially in the hours immediately after a rape. The directive seems to presume that there is a clear way to determine what the emergency contraceptive does, and thus ignores this practical issue. Daniel Sulmasy, a Catholic moralist and physician who supports the exception for rape victims, believes that there is still some scientific doubt about the precise mechanism of emergency contraception, even levonorgestrel. In his view, even the smallest likelihood of abortion ought to make Catholics wary. Thus, ideally, if it were possible to limit the use of emergency contraception to women who are neither ovulating nor already pregnant, then the possibility of harm to an embryo would be eliminated.

Because no test exists to determine conception in the earliest hours after intercourse, and since to be effective, emergency contraception must be administered within 72 hours of sex, it is virtually impossible to rule out whether a pregnancy has occurred. It is, however, possible to determine with some certainty whether a woman is in the ovulation phase of her cycle. If she is, then there is at least a likelihood that fertilization may have occurred. If she is not ovulating, then one could presume that fertilization has not occurred, and no embryo is endangered. Some Catholic hospitals have devised a thorough and systematized approach for determining whether the rape victim is ovulating or near the time of ovulation. This approach was developed in 1995 at Saint Francis Medical Center in Peoria, Illinois, and is now referred to as the "Peoria Protocol."[39] It consists of a test to determine whether or not a woman who has been raped is ovulating. If she is, then the hospital is not allowed to give her the emergency contraceptive because there is a small chance that a fertilized egg may be destroyed. This protocol raises a host of questions about the proper treatment of rape victims; yet many Catholic moralists see no problem in requiring the ovulation tests as a prerequisite for a woman to receive the emergency contraceptive.

The Peoria Protocol has been discussed, albeit briefly, in the pages of Catholic bioethics and health journals. Two camps have emerged— one that supports the use of methods to test for ovulation using the Peoria Protocol (dubbed the ovulation group), and one that holds that a pregnancy test is sufficient to determine whether it is safe to administer emergency contraception (the pregnancy group). What does the development of this protocol signify? On one hand, it could be seen as an attempt to support emergency contraception by silencing the critics who are concerned with its abortifacient effect. On the other hand, it certainly hinders accessibility to emergency contraception—putting rape victims through the additional trauma of determining the fact of whether or not they are ovulating would have the effect of discouraging them from using the pill. It is difficult at this point to know how seriously this debate will alter the overall trajectory of the Catholic view about emergency contraceptives, but it does suggest that Catholic acceptance of the scientific evidence about the mechanism of these contraceptives is at least possible.

We might also ask whether this directive reveals anything new about the Catholic discourses of contraception. On one hand, it seems to violate the Church's long-standing opposition to artificial contraception. Even if the evidence could show definitively that Plan B has no effect on an embryo, it still violates the Catholic teaching about the purposes and finality of the sexual act. On the other hand, it shows how violence and harm (rape in this case) are central features of the Catholic teaching about contraception, especially because of the persistent association of contraception with abortion. We see in this case, however, that the injustice of rape shifts the concern away from contraception per se toward self-defense against an unjust aggressor. The act of rape is not a proper sexual act, and thus interference with fertilization does not violate its natural structure.

To put the question more directly: Does dispensing emergency contraception to victims of sexual violence present us with an exception to the Catholic teaching on contraception? If so, what does that tell us about how exceptions function in Catholic moral thought? If not, why not? Determining what counts as an exception is deceptively difficult because often the terms of the argument are changed in order to accommodate a development in teaching. Thus, in this case, the official teaching deems that emergency contraception is not *really* contraception because rape is not *really* sex. Some moralists may want to view this as an exception in order to show that the Church's position on contraception is not immutable. Yet this question is further complicated because of the difficulty of how to characterize or describe this act—a difficulty that hangs on the distinction between the physical and moral aspects of the act. Is it contraceptive, both physically (i.e., in terms of its mechanism) and morally (i.e., in terms of the intent of the will of the agent)? The physical question, as I have already stated, is clouded by the Catholic belief that there is uncertainty about emergency contraception's mechanism: Does it prevent conception (contraceptive), or does it prevent implantation (abortifacient)? The moral question rests on two issues: (1) precision about the morally significant difference between rape and marital sexual intercourse; (2) precision about the difference in intention between one who is using emergency contraception and one who is using artificial contraception to prevent a pregnancy in marriage. Although it is easy to separate these two matters (the moral from the physical) in the abstract, we have seen that the Catholic discourse about contraception blurs the line between them. Clearly, the case of rape and emergency contraception tests the boundaries among sex, violence, and justice. Though sexual immorality was the central focus in the official Catholic response to the use of condoms for HIV/AIDS prevention, violence and injustice frame the matter of the use of emergency contraception for rape victims.

## The Historical Background of the Rape Exception

We can gain clarity on this matter by placing it in some historical context. Although the development of pharmaceutical emergency contraception is fairly recent, the question at the heart of the issue has received sustained attention from Catholic moralists since the seventeenth century, when moralists were concerned with the question "May a woman expel the semen of a rapist after an attack?" This question emerged in the context of another issue that was receiving much attention at the time: the matter of the *bimestre*—a two-month period immediately after a wedding during which, according to Canon Law, a woman could deny her husband sex. The idea was that a marriage that had not been sexually consummated could be dissolved easily, thereby allowing women time to contemplate the possibility of entering the convent and pursuing the religious life. The husband was also protected because this freed him to marry someone else soon after the dissolution of his marriage. The *bimestre* provided a way out of the marital duty, and it established a woman's right to refuse sex within marriage. This right had been established for other "intrinsic" reasons such as "drunkenness, insanity, serious disease, certain death from possible childbirth, nonsupport, etc."[40]

Moralists engaged in numerous debates about this two-month period when the wife could refuse sex. For example, they pondered the question of what might happen if a husband forced himself on his wife during this time. Would such an act constitute rape? And if so, would it be morally equivalent to rape outside of marriage? This question about whether a husband's forceful sexual insistence ought to be categorized as rape led moralists, most notably Thomas Sanchez, to ask whether the victim of a marital rape could justifiably expel the semen after intercourse. In other words, the attempt to decide the moral seriousness of forcing sex on one's wife during the *bimestre* led moralists to the question of contraception after rape.

Here is what Sanchez has to say about the matter: "May a wife forcefully violated by her husband before the two-month (*bimestre*) period is up expel the semen? It seems that she may not do so, because it is intrinsically evil and against nature, which orients the semen toward the propagation of offspring. But if we are speaking of a woman who has suffered violence, but not from her husband, I consider it certain: (1) that if she delays in expelling the semen, then she may not do so at all; but (2) if she expels the semen without delay, then it is strongly probable that she may licitly do this."[41]

Sanchez distinguishes between cases of forced sex within marriage and forced sex outside marriage. In the latter case, a woman may expel the semen as a way to avoid pregnancy, while in the former she may not. The reason for this distinction is the severity of the harm caused by each act. In Sanchez's view, the wife who is forced to have sex during the *bimestre* is not injured as seriously as the woman raped by someone other than her husband. He is particularly concerned with the injury to reputation sustained by a victim of extramarital rape. Notice that this view is connected to a premodern understanding of rape as forced sex on a woman who does "belong" to a man—a view that made the category of rape in marriage unintelligible.

Sanchez's position was controversial in his time. Other moralists held either that expulsion of semen was illicit in both cases or in neither. Mostly, however, Sanchez is remembered as a participant in the battles about probabilism, laxism, and rigorism in the seventeenth century. These doctrinal controversies were essentially about how to sort out the various opinions offered by moral theologians on difficult moral cases. Some held that if an opinion was probable—that is, corroborated by several moral authorities—it was then deemed authoritative. This led to tremendous abuses, which were famously addressed in Blaise Pascal's *Provincial Letters*. Bayer notes, however, that when Pope Innocent XI cracked down on Catholic casuists in 1679, he did not condemn Sanchez's doctrine regarding contraception and extramarital rape.[42]

As a result, Sanchez's teaching continued to be discussed and debated by moralists, most notably Saint Alphonsus Liguori in the early eighteenth century. Liguori was largely responsible for bringing order to moral theology in the aftermath of the laxist/rigorist controversies by proposing the position known as equiprobabilism.[43] This was an attempt to mark a middle path between the two extremes. On the issue of Sanchez's controversial view on the expulsion of semen after a rape, Liguori argues that the woman could legitimately resist the rapist, even if that led to "spilled semen," but once the semen had been deposited in the woman's body, she could not legitimately interfere with the physiological process. On the basis of an erroneous understanding of physiology, Liguori writes: "For immediately when the man ejaculates his semen (into the vagina) the matrix of the woman takes his semen up and encloses it within itself."[44]

Despite Liguori's prominence, Sanchez's position prevailed, at least to the extent that the Magisterium never officially condemned it in favor of Liguori's view; and by the early twentieth century, most moral theologians supported Sanchez's position on contraception after rape. It is difficult to know exactly what the basis of the contemporary position is, because most moralists simply cite the position as a given in the tradition without offering a detailed justification; but it appears to be based on a view that rape is not an authentic sexual act because the victim has not given her free consent. Thus the use of a contraceptive device in the context of such acts is not categorized as contraception; rather, it is the "prevention of pregnancy."[45] In this view, contraception is wrong not simply because it prevents pregnancy but because it involves a "contraceptive intention"—one that implies "an interior rejection of the substance of one's sexuality in its procreational dimension."[46]

Bayer argues that according to his reading of the Catholic tradition, a woman may also legitimately use *preventive* artificial contraception to avoid pregnancy in cases where her husband is forcing her (either physically or emotionally) to have sex. Bayer writes: "From such an act a woman can, in our view, justifiably seek to avoid pregnancy, not in positively performing a perverted act, but in negatively withholding a dimension of her sexuality, namely her fertility, *lest in surrendering that fertility, she compound the violence to which she is being subjected"* (emphasis added).[47]

A 1964 article by Felix Cardegna in *Theological Studies* provides us with a more contemporary treatment of how the then newly discovered birth control pill influenced moral deliberation on the issue of using contraception after a rape and also before an "anticipated" rape. Cardegna identifies what he sees as a gap or dissonance between the stated official teaching on artificial contraception and some of the "generally accepted solutions of Catholic casuistry." He claims that the Catholic teaching about contraception is absolute insofar as it is viewed as "a violation of the inviolable divine plan for the beginning of human life."[48] Nevertheless, moralists are always looking for ways to permit certain interventions. In his words, there are "a considerable number of intrusions into the inviolability of the conjugal act and the natural processes surrounding it."[49] Cardegna seeks to determine where Catholic moralists are drawing the line between what constitutes legitimate and illegitimate interferences with natural processes. He notes that the distinction between licit and illicit interference is usually characterized using the terms *accidental* and *substantial*—the former being licit and the latter illicit. Yet he concludes that this distinction lacks any true normative force or content: "These words give us no norm for deciding which interventions go too far to be permitted."[50] In other words, the terms are essentially empty.

Cardegna suggests that the more helpful distinction is one between acts that interfere with the natural structure of the marital act and those that interfere with the reproductive process. The minimal requirement for a marital act, according to Catholic teaching, is the depositing of the male's sperm into the female's vagina.[51] Hence any interference with the natural structure (condoms, barrier methods) transforms the physical act such that it can no longer be considered a marital act; it has lost its integrity.[52] Actions that intrude into the generative biological processes (sterilization) alter the process of generation, while not changing the physical components of the sexual act. Thus, sterilization, which does not interfere with the marriage act (the sperm still can reach its final destination) but clearly alters the generative faculty, is perhaps a less serious violation. This view that sterilization might be morally less serious than barrier methods provides Cardegna with an opening to argue for the possible acceptance of the birth control pill.

Cardegna also discusses examples that test the line between licit and illicit interference in the generative process. One licit practice at the time was the use of drugs to suppress sexual desire with the intention to limit the size of a family. Another was the use of the birth control pill by women who were breast-feeding and wanted to ensure that their ovulation was suppressed. Cardegna claims that this practice was not considered a form of forbidden sterilization because it was not interfering with "*normal*" fertility because "ovulation during the lactation period is considered to be abnormal fertility."[53] We shall return to this case later in the chapter in our discussion of exceptional cases. Such cases reinforce Cardegna's view that the distinction between contraceptives that interfere with the structure of the act and those that merely interfere with the generative process is a valid one.

Cardegna also contemplates cases of women who used contraception following a rape, along with cases of women who, in danger of being raped, used contraceptive devices preemptively.[54] He analyzes the views of the moralists John C. Ford and Gerald Kelly, who defend the use of contraceptives by raped women. They argue that because raped women do not will intercourse, they can licitly will "the frustration of the natural purpose of the act." In other words, what is immoral about contraception is that one wills to have sexual intercourse while willing that conception does not occur. These, according to Ford and Kelly, are "contradictory acts of the will." A woman who has been raped would not experience this contradiction because she is merely willing one thing—that she not conceive. Ford and Kelly's view on this point was not held by all moralists. Some continued to argue that all contraception was illicit because it interfered with the *physiological* process of generation. But as noted above, Cardegna does not agree. He embraces a morally relevant distinction between interference with the physical structure of the act and interference with the process of generation.

Clearly, Ford and Kelly held a decidedly progressive view on this issue.[55] They recognized that rape was not a sexual act (insofar as the woman is not willing it), and thus any action to prevent conception in such a case would not violate the totality and finality of sexual intercourse. Thus, in a technical sense, they were claiming that a raped woman who frustrates conception is not really engaged in contraception. They even asserted that "contraceptive acts are absolutely forbidden, but we are not always clear whether a given act is contraceptive."[56]

As with Sanchez and others before them, they did not intend their justification for allowing contraception after a rape to be an exception. Rather, they redefined the act, and in doing so moved the conversation from the realm of sexual ethics to the ethics of just responses to aggression.

This justification continues to be supported by some contemporary theologians. For example, Germain Grisez, whose views about condom use were discussed in the previous chapter, makes a similar argument. He claims that artificial contraception can be used to prevent a pregnancy resulting from rape. He even goes as far as to state that even "a slight risk of abortion" can be "accepted as a side effect."[57] This position is surprising in light of Grisez's long-standing rejection of contraceptive use, even to protect the life of a woman. Interestingly, here he is concerned with "a defense of the woman's ovum (insofar as it is a part of her person) against the rapist's sperms (insofar as they are parts of his person)."[58] However, any direct use of an abortifacient would be illicit. A case of rape is unlike the case of intercourse "sought out or willingly permitted" by the woman, because her intention is clear: there is no contradiction. Grisez holds that when one engages in sexual intercourse willingly (and he has a pretty loose definition of what constitutes willingness), then any prevention of conception is a choice against life.[59]

## Rape in Catholic Teaching

These moralists' comfort with changing the terms of the discussion suggests that it is important to situate these terms in their historic contexts. One such term is "rape," a topic that has received relatively little direct scholarly attention from Catholic moralists. As for official Vatican statements, it is only recently that they have framed the topic as one related to the oppression of women. Interestingly, ecclesiastical law defines rape as a grave sin against chastity that also does harm to justice and charity.[60] Thus, it is primarily a sexual sin—a position that is strikingly different from the view of the moralists discussed above, who view rape as violence rather than as sex. This definition also leaves open the question of whose chastity is violated, the rapist's or the victim's? One can presume that it is primarily in reference to the rapist's, but that is not at all explicit or clear in the definition. As we shall see, there is a strong tradition in Catholicism of rape narratives where the victim dies while resisting rape in order to protect her chastity. Thomas Aquinas categorized rape as a species of lust, along with fornication, seduction, incest, adultery, sacrilege, and "the sin against nature." "The sin of lust," he wrote, "consists in seeking venereal pleasure not in accordance with right reason." This can occur in two ways: by being inconsistent with the natural end of the act, or by involving another person with whom one is not in right relation (incest is the misuse of a woman to whom one is related; adultery and seduction consist of having sexual relations with a woman who is not under a man's authority). Rape is connected to seduction, in that it involves sex with a woman who is under the authority of her father, but with the added dimension of violence. In other words, much of the evil of the act comes from a man having sex with a woman over whom he has no authority.[61] This way of characterizing rape connects it to the Seventh Commandment concerning stealing and justice.

Thus, although the tradition has always recognized the injustice of using physical violence to force a woman to have sex against her will, it was also concerned with the effect of rape on a woman's chastity, along with the injustice it brought to the individual who had authority over her. Over time, however, these views have become less explicit in the official teaching. For example, the Thomistic emphasis on rape as a violation of a person over whom one has no authority was replaced by an emphasis on the dignity of women and the need to respect them as persons. Note the following passage from Pope John Paul II's 1995 "Letter to Women": "The time has come to condemn vigorously the types of *sexual violence* which frequently have women for their object and to pass laws which effectively defend them from such violence. Nor can we fail, in the name of the respect due to the human person, to condemn the widespread hedonistic and commercial culture which encourages the systematic exploitation of sexuality and corrupts even very young girls into letting their bodies be used for profit."[62]

In this passage, the pope acknowledges the existence of violence against women, but he emphasizes that it was a problem that existed in the public sphere and was in need of a public remedy: more laws to defend women against violence. He also identifies the source of such violence in peaceful and prosperous societies as "hedonistic permissiveness" that "aggravates tendencies to aggressive male behavior." Such an assertion contradicts much feminist analysis of rape, which views unjust patriarchal power structures as primarily responsible for male aggression. The passage also omits any mention of whether rape is a violation of chastity. After identifying the problem and diagnosing its cause, the pope turns specifically to the issue of abortion in cases of rape:[63]

> In contrast to these sorts of perversion, what great appreciation must be shown to those women who, with a heroic love for the child they have conceived, proceed with a pregnancy resulting from the injustice of rape. Here we are thinking of atrocities perpetrated not only in situations of war, still so common in the world, but also in societies which are blessed by prosperity and peace and yet are often corrupted by a culture of hedonistic permissiveness which aggravates tendencies to aggressive male behaviour. In these cases the choice to have an abortion always remains a grave sin. But before being something to blame on the woman, it is a crime for which guilt needs to be attributed to men and to the complicity of the general social environment.[64]

Here, he not only reiterates the Catholic prohibition of abortion in such cases but also uses the opportunity to commend women who continue with such pregnancies. Their heroic love for the child overrides any anguish that may come from bearing a child who is the result of rape.

From this lengthy discussion of the issue by Pope John Paul II, one can see that rape figures prominently in the context of two larger issues in Catholic moral teaching: concern about overly permissive sexual cultures and abortion. The connection between rape and oppressive gender structures is not mentioned. This blindness to the connection is especially evident in the most common forum for Catholic discourse about rape: stories of heroic women who are willing to die rather than be raped. Christianity is rife with such stories; indeed, the narratives of early Christian martyrdom were modeled precisely on the idea of a defense of virginity. Even in the context of the past two centuries, the Vatican has used the virgin/martyr story to reiterate the centrality of the virtue of chastity in the context of rape. For example, in a speech commemorating the centennial of the death of Saint Maria Goretti, Pope John Paul II characterized her death at the hands of the man who attempted to rape her as exemplifying a love of chastity that stands in sharp contrast to "a culture that idolizes the physical aspect of the relations between a man and a woman."[65] The pope did not view the attempted rape of this young girl as an opportunity to address the issue of rape per se.[66] Rather, it was an opportunity for him to hold her up as an example of someone who held fast to God's commandments. He stated: "She did not break God's commandment in spite of being threatened by death."[67]

It is interesting to juxtapose this perspective on rape and martyrdom with the definition of rape as an intrinsically evil act in the *Catechism*. Is the implication that if Goretti had not successfully resisted, then her act would have been the intrinsically evil one? This way of viewing the virgin/martyr is typical of Christian accounts that depict her as having given her life to avoid committing an intrinsic evil. Thus, these narratives seem to suggest that there are two possible "intrinsically evil acts" in instances of rape; the act of the rapist, and the lack of sufficient resistance on the part of the victim. This places the burden of resistance on the victim, not only as a way to protect her bodily safety, but also as a way to protect her moral standing. Most Catholic sources confirm that a woman who is being raped is expected to resist. They draw a distinction between external and internal resistance. The internal concerns the will insofar as a woman is never to consent to the rape with her will. As for external resistance, she is expected to resist physically as much as possible, "without endangering her life or reputation."[68] For our purposes, however, it clarifies the discourse surrounding the use of contraceptives after rape as a type of resistance or response to violence. The victim is allowed to continue resisting her aggressor, even after the rape, by destroying or blocking the sperm's ability to fertilize her egg. The morality of the emergency contraceptive is judged through the framework of violence. It is not viewed as centrally connected to the problem of sexual immorality in an individual.[69] Thus the moral understanding of rape shifts in the context of resistance.

The matter of what constitutes adequate resistance is a bit murky in Catholic teaching. Most famously, Saint Augustine addresses the question of the effect of rape on a victim's sexual and moral purity. He raises this issue in the context of a broader discussion of suicide and whether a woman who commits suicide as a way to prevent a rape or in reaction to the shame of having been raped is in fact committing homicide. He concludes that she was, and bases this on the idea that purity resides in the will, because though humans can control their wills, they do not always have control over their bodies. To illustrate his point, he gives the example of the case of a midwife who accidentally (or even maliciously) destroys the virginity of a girl "while endeavoring to ascertain it." In such a case, Augustine claims, the harm to the girl's body in no way compromises the integrity of her soul. He writes: "So long as the soul keeps this firmness of purpose which sanctifies even the body, the violence done by another's lust makes no impression on this bodily sanctity, which is preserved intact by one's own persistent continence."[70] Contemporary martyr stories like Goretti's send the message that surviving rape is not desirable and perhaps even a violation of God's commandments. She preferred death over the violation of her chastity. By contrast, Augustine is firm in claiming that the victim's purity can remain intact and that she is no way guilty or responsible for what happened to her.[71]

## Preemptive Contraception: Taking Steps to Prevent Pregnancy before a Rape

We turn now to a different type of case—one that involves the use of contraceptives before the fact; that is, in cases where there is a threat of rape. This issue of preemptive contraception was debated vigorously by Catholic moralists in the early 1960s. The case that then received much attention in the pages of Catholic journals was that of the Catholic nuns in the Belgian Congo.[72] Ambrogio Valsecchi describes this "test" case in general terms: "It is the case of a woman, more precisely of a nun, who, fearing she may be raped makes use of progestational drugs to induce sterility and prevent any eventual conception."[73] Bayer also recounts the case and provides a little more detail about "the plight of religious Sisters and other women caught up in the uprisings in the Belgian Congo." He writes: "These women were given anovulant drugs by doctors on the missions in order to ward off pregnancy which might otherwise result from the rape which was a constant threat in that chaotic episode." Bayer also described the Magisterium's lack of response to this issue. He claims that "the Magisterium, however, made no effort to intervene . . . and . . . even quietly reviewed the case and tacitly accepted the actions of the mission doctors as being in harmony with the moral doctrine of the Church."[74] Valsecchi does not conclude that the discussions that emerged from this case, and in particular the solution proposed, "formed the point of transition to a new manner of considering the whole question of progestational drugs."[75] Yet Cardegna, in his article discussed above, sees the use of preemptive contraception as an example of the gap between official teaching and sanctioned practices.

Valsecchi summarizes the opinions of various authors who wrote about the case, pointing out the use of the principles of double effect and totality in their arguments. He discusses two authors who concluded that the pill can be used licitly in this case. They rely on various arguments, all of which involve the question of the women's intention. For instance, one author, P. Palazzini, claims that the temporary sterilization caused by the pill is indirect "inasmuch as 'the intention of the procedure is not the interruption of ovulation but the prevention of the consequences of an eventual violation of chastity.'" He further claims that the use of the pill in this case is licit because the motivation is to calm the fear and anguish of the woman and to preserve "the present and future physical and psychical well-being of the woman."[76] Joseph Farraher, SJ, also reviews this debate about the use of contraception in the rape defense test case, and he concludes that the action could be licit. He describes his argument as follows: "The act is certainly a direct sterilization and is contraceptive in intent, but in the circumstances does not contain the evil for which sterilization and contraception are generally sinful."[77] Interestingly, Farraher does not consider the categories of object of the act and intention as relevant to this case. The circumstances of the act are what change the nature of the act and render it licit. You will recall that Cardegna, following Ford and Kelly, claims contraception is immoral because it is contradictory for the agent to will to have sexual intercourse and to will to avoid conception in the same act. Because the rape victim does not will to have sexual intercourse, her act is not contradictory and thus not contraceptive. On this view, the person who uses contraception to prevent pregnancy when they do not will the sexual act is engaged in a radically different act from the person who wills the sexual act but does not will the resulting pregnancy. As noted by Farraher, the intention in both cases is contraceptive, but the sinfulness of contraception is based on the evil of wanting to experience sexual pleasure while avoiding its possible consequence.

Unlike Goretti, who was resisting the rape, the nuns were resisting the possibility of a pregnancy. The discussions in journals of moral theology focus on whether or not it was licit for the nuns to avoid pregnancy, rather than on their resistance to rape. Indeed, based on the logic of Goretti's canonization, one might ask why these nuns did not die resisting their rapists.[78] Implicit in their request for the pill is a sense that though the rape cannot be prevented, at the very least a pregnancy might be prevented. This is in stark contrast to the earlier history of virgin/martyrs who, either because they would commit suicide or allow themselves to be killed before being raped, might not have worried about the possibility of a pregnancy.

Jane Tibbetts Schulenburg has written about various strategies employed by medieval nuns living under the threat of rape. She discusses cloistering and suicide, but also raises a third type of response—the *virginitas deformitate* defense, the practice of self-mutilation.[79] Although not identical, there are interesting parallels between this response and the case of preemptive contraception. Schulenburg discusses accounts of groups of cloistered nuns, who under imminent threat of rape would mutilate their faces as a way to scare off potential attackers. This mode of "virginal self-defense," though difficult to corroborate historically, does serve to emphasize the lengths to which virgins would go to protect their purity. In the contemporary case, the nuns considering contraception were clearly thinking in a radically different way about what they were defending and preventing.

Here again, we confront the problem of how to describe and organize the moral categories that frame rape and contraception. Seeing these acts as violations of chastity limits our vision and perpetuates the idea that acts of rape are sexual acts. Clearly, the category of violence or harm to life is the most relevant one here. Yet the Catholic discourses of martyrdom and resistance to rape present mixed messages as they move back and forth between the categories of sins against chastity, against life, and against justice. Finally, in the contemporary context, the framework of justice might be the most promising for understanding the morality of Catholic hospitals and emergency contraception. The use of contraceptives either before or after a rape can be seen as an application of the ideal of justice and fairness. If the sperm of the rapist is an "unjust" aggressor, then the victim is morally entitled to respond.

## THE PROHIBITION AGAINST CONTRACEPTION AND DIFFICULT CASES

The birth control pill was the subject of great scrutiny in the decade leading up to *Humanae vitae*. The history of the early Catholic reactions to its use contributes to understanding the background of the contemporary view. As is the case with Plan B, much of the debate among moral theologians focused on the uncertainty surrounding the biological mechanism of the pill. More specifically, moralists were debating whether or not the pill's intervention was "natural." John Rock, one of the developers of the birth control pill and a Catholic, was arguing at the time that the pill did not violate Catholic principles because "the oral contraceptive simply duplicates the action of this [progesterone] natural hormone when the woman herself feels the necessity for protection of her young—present or prospective."[80] The Catholic moralist John Lynch, SJ, rejects Rock's argument, claiming that in addition to ignoring the Church's teaching on direct sterilization, it is illogical. He argues that not all interventions in natural processes are licit; for example, death is natural, but we would not sanction anyone who would intervene to bring it about. More relevant to our discussion is an internal debate about whether the pill can be used in cases where the direct intention was not contraceptive. Lynch concludes that on the basis of the principle of double effect, some uses could be allowed, such as for regularizing menstrual cycles. Pope Pius XII had ruled in 1958 that this was a legitimate use of the pill—a view that was confirmed by Pope Paul VI in *Humanae vitae* a decade later.[81] Lynch asserts: "Only when it is evident that some genuine malady requires the remedial effects of the drugs in question can we begin to think and speak in terms of an indirect suppression of generative function which may be allowed for sufficiently serious reason."[82]

Although the indirect effect of contraception that might result from using the pill to treat menstrual irregularities was deemed acceptable, Lynch finds other cases more challenging. He discusses two in particular. One concerns women who might use the pill for a few months to regularize their cycle so that they would be able to practice natural family planning more effectively. The other concerns women who wanted to avoid pregnancy in the postpartum period, a case discussed earlier by Cardegna. For most women, breast-feeding ensures that ovulation is halted, which leads to a form of temporary sterility that has traditionally allowed women to space out the births of their children. Lynch poses the following question about this case: "In the event, however, that nature should fail—as at least sometimes it does—to provide this period of natural sterility, can justification be found for using the pills in order to insure oneself against the 'accident' of ovulation which, through nature's oversight as it were, might otherwise occur?"[83]

Some moralists were arguing that in cases of women where this natural function is not working, the pill can provide them with a kind of protection that ought to be theirs naturally. Lynch is not convinced by that argument. He worries greatly about the difficulty of determining what ought to count as normal functioning of a woman's generative process. He distinguishes cases where the pill was being used as a remedy "for certain serious anomalies of menstruation" from those where it was used to regulate menstruation for the express purpose of helping the couple practice the rhythm method of family planning more effectively. In the first type of case, a woman's health and well-being are affected by the menstrual irregularity, whereas in the second type of case, the intention is not as obviously therapeutic. Lynch concedes that "there is a sharp difference of opinion among theologians" on this issue. They are divided on the issue of whether the temporary sterility caused by the pill is "the directly intended means whereby regularity of ovulation is accomplished" or whether it is "an indirect by-product of therapy whose direct result is regularization of the ovulatory cycle."[84]

Richard McCormick offers another perspective on this issue. Building on Lynch's position, he distinguishes three types of antifertility medication: (1) those that achieve a temporary state of sterility, (2) those whose purpose is abortifacient, and (3) those that cause temporary sterility but have other effects as well. The first type, according to McCormick, is absolutely forbidden because it violates both the Fifth Commandment and Sixth Commandment. Although the violation of the Sixth Commandment is obvious from a Catholic perspective (temporary sterility would enable individuals to pursue "unchaste" sex), the violation of the Fifth Commandment is a little more ambiguous. Temporary sterility violates the Fifth Commandment because it is considered an "illicit mutilation," a point to which Lynch alluded earlier. McCormick writes: "Mutilation is, generally speaking, any action whereby an organic function or the distinctive use of any member is suppressed or notably diminished." Now, according to Church teaching, not all mutilation is illicit; it is licit when performed for the greater good of the whole person, as in the case of a life-saving surgical procedure. But the "human generative faculty" is different because "men are endowed with generative ability not primarily for their personal benefit, but for the good of the very species." Thus, directly acting to cause temporary sterility is an act against the common good of the species.[85]

The second type is prohibited for the same reasons that abortion is prohibited, namely, the intentional destruction of a human life—a violation of the Fifth Commandment. The third category is the one that raises the most interesting questions for our purposes. This type of act involves cases where temporary sterility is a foreseen but not directly intended consequence. So, for example, although the agent knows that temporary sterility will result from taking the birth control pill, her intention in doing so might be to treat a menstrual irregularity. The temporary sterility itself is not a means for achieving her desired end, but, to use McCormick's language, simply a by-product of the act. Under the category of this third type of potentially ambiguous acts, McCormick describes five difficult cases (some real and some hypothetical) with which Catholic moralists were dealing in the early 1960s.[86] These were (1) the correction of menstrual disorders, (2) the ovulation rebound, (3) delaying menstruation, (4) the suppression of ovulation during lactation, and (5) the regularization of the menstrual cycle to improve the efficacy of rhythm method. Of these five scenarios, the first two were considered licit by most commentators. The first case involved the use of the birth control pill to help women with menstrual symptoms that stem from certain physical disorders. According to McCormick, moralists distinguish between two aspects of ovarian function—the generative and the endocrine. As long as the intention of the agent is to affect the latter and not the former, then all is well. The temporary sterility that would result is viewed as an unintended or indirect effect of the primary intended act. Here the birth control pill is viewed as a therapeutic treatment aimed at repairing the ovaries' endocrine function.

The other noncontroversial case was the potential use of the pill to help a sterile woman regain her fertility.[87] McCormick notes that, in the view of most commentators, the woman's status as sterile or infertile meant that the pill did not have a contraceptive effect; nor was it the agent's intention to use it for this purpose. Although generating some controversy, the third case of women using the pill to delay menstruation because of an important event (McCormick gives the example of an important sporting event) was a relatively simple one for most moralists. Because there was no contraceptive intent and because ovulation was merely delayed rather than suppressed, most moralists approved of this use. McCormick notes one contrary argument that raises the question of whether this action could be deemed therapeutic. If the action is not therapeutic, then it is in violation of the principle of totality, which claims that a mutilation of the body (and chemical sterilization is considered to be mutilation in most official Catholic accounts) is illicit unless undertaken for a greater good.

The matter of whether the use of a contraceptive is therapeutic is clearly the most important consideration in sorting out the two remaining difficult cases. As we have noted, whether an action is intended or merely foreseen is a critical distinction in Catholic moral theology.[88] Thus, in cases that are primarily therapeutic, at least in intent, the action is licit as long as it does not interfere with the physical structure of the act. The case involving regularizing a menstrual cycle for the purpose of a more accurate use of the rhythm method is interesting in this regard, because much of the discussion involved determining whether an irregular menstrual cycle was pathological or abnormal. If one could make the case that it was, then using the pill to address the abnormality might make it licit. Of course, the problem of intention still lingers in this case, as it seems fairly obvious that a woman would not actively address this pathology unless her ultimate goal was contraceptive. McCormick states that most moralists approved of this because it was a therapeutic and thus indirect sterilization.

The final interesting case that McCormick highlights is the one both Cardegna and Lynch discuss: the use of the pill by women who are breast-feeding. Here again, the argument rests on whether one could support the claim that women who ovulate while breast-feeding are suffering from a pathological condition that ought to be remedied. McCormick notes some practical difficulties associated with such a case. In agreement with Lynch, he points to the difficulty of determining exactly the precise moment when ovulation becomes abnormal. Moreover, he notes that this reasoning could apply to premenopausal women whose ovulation is irregular. As in the previous case, most moralists conclude that the intention is ultimately contraceptive—there really is no other benefit.

McCormick's discussion of these cases helps us to distill some key points in understanding the history of Catholic conversations about artificial contraception and how those might have an impact on the specific issue of this chapter, emergency contraception for victims of rape. First, though Catholic evaluations often appeal to the distinction of intended versus foreseen consequences of an act, that distinction is not relevant to the case of emergency contraception in cases of rape.

Contraception is clearly the direct intention; but as we have seen, Catholic moralists believe that the circumstance of the act changes the nature of the act sufficiently so that contraception is now viewed as a defense against injustice. Second, these difficult cases that McCormick discusses often rely on the distinction between therapeutic and non-therapeutic intervention. Although the contemporary discussion of emergency contraception does not rely on this distinction, it is still worth thinking about how it could clarify matters. Emergency contraception does bring about a temporary sterilization, which traditionally has been considered an act of mutilation. In the cases discussed above, mutilation is allowed only when the overall good of the organism requires it. The overall good has generally been construed rather narrowly as the physical, rather than psychic, good. In the case of rape victims, however, the good is construed much more broadly. In fact, the language of injustice extends it to encompass a more communal sense of the good.

## CONCLUSION

The issues raised by emergency contraception in the case of rape are significant. I began the chapter by posing a set of questions about the US Catholic bishops' decision to sanction the use of emergency contraception for rape victims—at least in principle. I asked how this decision fit into the tradition's long-standing refusal to allow for the use of artificial contraceptives. Is it an exception to an otherwise absolute prohibition? And if so, do they justify it on the basis of concerns about justice? Do these concerns eclipse the rhetoric of chastity and the objective moral order? From a feminist perspective, viewing the use of contraceptives by rape victims as an altogether different act reinforces the important point that rape is not a sexual act—it is an act of violence. Yet in the context of the Catholic discourse about rape, where this insight is not sufficiently developed, the force of the distinction is weakened.

This position appears to affirm that the moral evaluation of contraception only makes sense in the context of sexual acts. Rape is a different species of act; thus interfering with the natural outcome of rape is significantly different than interfering with an act of marital intercourse. The tradition describes rape as an inauthentic sexual act and therefore not naturally ordained to certain ends. Contraception taken after rape is not interference with the natural order; the act of rape itself is a violation of the objective moral order, an intrinsically evil act. The rape victim's decision to use emergency contraception is not one based in concerns about her chastity because she is not in a position to think about "the successful integration" of her sexuality. Indeed, rape is ultimately an act that dis-integrates the victim. The language of chastity is thus not particularly helpful in thinking about how to respond to rape. The language of chastity is of limited use in justifying the use of emergency contraception for a rape victim. Perhaps the same limitations may apply in all cases of contraception. Although chastity draws attention to the central role of integrity in Catholic sexual ethics, it remains too individualistic a virtue to address the broader implications that are better captured by the category of justice. Justice, by contrast, does provide ways to think about and respond to the act of rape. How contraception matters to the common good is the primary topic of concern for population and development issues, to which we turn in the next chapter.

## NOTES

1. For a careful discussion of what the term "intrinsic evil" does and does not mean, see Kaveny, "Intrinsic Evil." Kaveny draws attention to the way the term has been appropriated as part of prophetic discourse in Catholic circles, when in fact, its roots are firmly casuistic. She also emphasizes that the term does not "say anything about the comparative gravity of the act." In other words, there are cases of acts that are not intrinsically evil (e.g., war) that are more serious evils than intrinsically evil acts (e.g, masturbation).

2. Office of Population Affairs, "Emergency Contraception Fact Sheet."

3. According to the National Conference of State Legislatures, in 2011 "Secretary of the Department of Health and Human Services Kathleen Sibelius disagreed with the FDA's decision [to provide over-the-counter access to girls under seventeen] and Plan B One-Step remains available for all ages, but still requires a prescription for women under the age of 17."

4. The birth control pill was first approved by the FDA in 1960. For a history of the development of the pill, see Watkins, *On the Pill*. Also, on a historical note, Noonan cites historical evidence of postcoital potions from documents as early as the fourth century CE; Noonan, *Contraception*, 13–14.

5. Coeytaux and Pillsbury, "Bringing Emergency Contraception to American Women," 80.

6. The FDA approved Searle's application to market Enovid as a contraceptive in 1960, but limited its prescription to one year or less. Watkins, *On the Pill*, 32.

7. For an interesting account of the early debates about possible dangers of the pill, see Watkins, *On the Pill*, chap. 4, "Debating the Safety of the Pill."

8. Coeytaux and Pillsbury, "Bringing Emergency Contraception to American Women," 81.

9. Ibid.

10. Faúndes et al., "Emergency Contraception," 131. The Yuzpe regimen identified several already-approved hormonal oral contraceptives that could be used in combination. For a brief period in the late 1990s, the FDA approved a dedicated product that combined the two hormones. It was marketed under the name Preven. It was discontinued once research indicated that levonorgestrel, used alone, was more effective; Murphy, "Update on Emergency Contraception."

11. Sanfilippo and Downing, "Emergency Contraception," 1.

12. Wood, Drazen, and Greene, "Politics of Emergency Contraception," 101–2.

13. Brunton and Beal, "Current Issues," 458.

14. One area of concern about long-acting contraception that drew much attention in those early decades was the racist subtext behind many efforts to force poor women, many of whom were women of color, to use these contraceptives. See Roberts, *Killing the Black Body*, esp. chap. 3.

15. Sanfilippo and Downing, "Emergency Contraception," 132.

16. Gemzell-Danielsson, Berger, and Lalitkumar, "Emergency Contraception," 305.

17. Wood, Drazen, and Greene, "Politics of Emergency Contraception," 101.

18. Watkins's discussion of the divisions in the 1960s about whether the pill or the IUD would be most effective for large-scale population control points to the politicized nature of many of the debates about birth control. In particular, she describes how the IUD was "depicted as birth control for the masses" and championed primarily by "international population controllers." Watkins, *On the Pill*, 70–71. Mifepristone is an antiprogestogen—i.e., a progesterone receptor blocker.

19. Murphy, "Update on Emergency Contraception," 599.

20. Brunton and Beal, "Current Issues," 459.

21. Glasier, "Emergency Contraception," 310.

22. Von Hertzen and Van Look, "Research on New Methods," 53.

23. Pontifical Academy for Life, "Statement."

24. This view explains the Catholic opposition to stem cell research, along with one of its reasons for opposing some reproductive technologies.

25. Pontifical Academy for Life, "Statement," par. 6.

26. Pontifical Academy for Life, "Final Declaration."

27. This instruction was issued under William Cardinal Levada, the prefect of the Congregation for the Doctrine of Faith, and was approved by Pope Benedict XVI. Congregation for the Doctrine of Faith, *Dignitas personae*.

28. Ibid., par. 23.

29. See the detailed discussion given by Noonan, *Contraception*, esp. 65–106.

30. Sulmasy, "Emergency Contraception," 309.

31. Croxatto and Diaz Fernandez, "Emergency Contraception," 312.

32. Sulmasy, "Emergency Contraception," 309.

33. US Conference of Catholic Bishops, *Ethical and Religious Directives.*

34. National Conference of State Legislatures, "50-State Summary." The states are Arkansas, California, Colorado, Connecticut, Illinois, Massachusetts, Minnesota, New Jersey, New Mexico, New York, Oregon, South Carolina, Texas, Utah, Washington, and Wisconsin.

35. Hamel and Panicola, "Emergency Contraception," 12–19.

36. *Christian Century*, "Morning-After Pill OK," 577.

37. Sulmasy, "Emergency Contraception."

38. Tonti-Filippini and Walsh, "Postcoital Intervention," 288.

39. For a description, see Hamel and Panicola, "Emergency Contraception and Sexual Assault."

40. Bayer, *Rape*, 14.

41. Thomas Sanchez, SJ, *Disputationes de Sancto Matrimonio* (Antuerpiae, 1624); quoted by Bayer, *Rape*, 15. In Bayer's discussion of this quotation, he notes that although Sanchez commonly used other writers (both from the past and contemporary to him) to corroborate his positions on moral points, he does not do so on this issue. This leads Bayer to assert that "as far as we can tell, he [Sanchez] is raising these questions for the first time in the history of Catholic moral theology"; Bayer, *Rape*, 15.

42. Bayer, *Rape*, 22–24.

43. For a discussion of the role of probabilism in Catholic moral theology, see Mahoney, *Making of Moral Theology*, 135–43.

44. This discussion of Sanchez and Liguori and the debate about probabilism is taken from Bayer, *Rape*, 33.

45. Ibid., 4–6.

46. Ibid., 5.

47. Ibid., 9.

48. Cardegna, "Contraception," 612.

49. Ibid.

50. Ibid., 615.

51. This argument is used by Germain Grisez, as seen in the previous chapter on condoms and HIV/AIDS.

52. Cardegna, "Contraception," 624.

53. Ibid., 614.

54. "Then there are the cases of rape which seem to allow a woman direct dominion over her reproductive faculties in special circumstances. A woman who has been raped is allowed to take contraceptive measures after the event. In cases of danger of rape, she is allowed to use a contraceptive diaphragm. And lately the opinion has been accepted which would allow her to take sterilizing drugs in such circumstances"; ibid., 613.

55. It is important to remember that Ford and Kelly were generally not "liberal" or "progressive" in their views about contraception. For an in-depth study of Ford's theological contributions, see Genilo, *John Cuthbert Ford.*

56. Ford and Kelly, 367–68, quoted by Cardegna, "Contraception," 615.

57. Grisez, *Way of the Lord Jesus*, 512n103.

58. Ibid.

59. Grisez writes, "Contraception always involves a choice to impede new human life: life is one of the basic human goods; the seventh and eighth modes of responsibility exclude choosing to impede any of the basic human goods. So, contraception is always wrong." Ibid., 512–13.

60. The *Catechism* states: "Rape is the forcible violation of the sexual intimacy of another person. It does injury to justice and charity. Rape deeply wounds the respect, freedom, and physical and moral integrity to which every person has a right. It causes grave damage that can mark the victim for life. It is always an intrinsically evil act. Graver still is the rape of children committed by parents (incest) or those responsible for the education of the children entrusted to them." *Catechism of the Catholic Church*, par. 2356.

61. Thomas Aquinas, *Summa Theologiae*, II. II., q. 154, art. 7. Thomas viewed all the sins that comprise the species of lust as sins against the virtue of chastity, which is a virtue related to temperance.

62. John Paul II, "Letter to Women," par. 5.

63. He does not mention the use of emergency contraception after a rape, probably because in 1995 such chemical interventions were not widely available.

64. John Paul II, "Letter to Women," par. 5.

65. John Paul II, "Maria Goretti."

66. Most accounts of her rape claim that she was twelve years old when Alessandro Serenelli (sometimes described as a neighbor and sometimes as a farmhand) attempted to rape her. She is reported to have cried out in the midst of the attempted rape, "No! It is a sin! God does not want it!" He then is said to have stabbed her fourteen times in anger over her resistance. She was found by her family and rushed to a neighboring town, where physicians tried to save her life. Her biographers claim that "after 20 painful hours of suffering, during which she forgave and prayed for Alessandro," she died. "Saint Maria Goretti Biography," www.ma riagoretti.org/mariabio.htm.

67. Ibid.

68. Hardon, *Modern Catholic Dictionary*.

69. The Church's rhetoric about rape is often connected to a critique of sexually permissive and immoral culture, as in the case of Maria Goretti.

70. Saint Augustine, *City of God*, book 1, chap. 18.

71. Anne Patrick refers to Catholic narratives that privilege "the patriarchal paradigm of virtue" as narratives "with fading power." Patrick contrasts her positive childhood and adolescent memories of Maria Goretti's sainthood with her feminist revulsion at the papal discourse about another contemporary virgin martyr, Saint Marie Clementine Anwarite, who was beatified by Pope John Paul II in 1985. Patrick raises similar concerns about patriarchal views of rape and virginity that would suggest that virginity is more important than life itself. Patrick, "Narrative and the Social Dynamics of Virtue," 84–88.

72. Sexual violence perpetrated on women who are by definition not sexually active is an odd place to begin discussions about whether using the pill is licit. In recent years, long after the heated internal debates of the 1960s, a Spanish bishop argued that nuns who live in war zones, where they might be susceptible to rape, ought to be allowed to use the pill. This appears once again to be the one exception that some Catholic priests feel comfortable suggesting. Thus, women who are intentionally not sexualized are viewed as safe exceptions, because there is no relationship between contraception and their sexual desires.

73. Valsecchi, *Controversy*, 26.

74. Bayer, *Rape*, 82–83.

75. Valsecchi, *Controversy*, 26.

76. Ibid., 27–28.

77. Farraher, "Notes," 85.

78. I realize that our ability to answer such a question is limited by the lack of information we have about the precise situations these nuns faced.

79. Schulenburg, *Forgetful of Their Sex*, 145.

80. Rock, "We Can End the Battle," quoted by Lynch, "Notes," 240.

81. *Humanae vitae*, par. 15.

82. Lynch, "Notes," 247.

83. Ibid., 245.

84. Ibid., 244.

85. McCormick, "Anti-Fertility Pills."

86 We have already seen this discussed by Lynch and Cardegna.

87. This notion that the pill could actually help infertile women regain their fertility is no longer considered sound. In fact, most studies in recent decades have focused on whether the pill has a long-term negative impact on women's fertility. One exception is a recent study that showed that women who used the pill actually had a higher chance of conceiving. See Farrow et al., "Prolonged Use."

88. For more on this, see Kaczor, *Edge of Life*, 67–81.

# CHAPTER 5

# JUSTICE

## Population, Development, and the Common Good

I N 1965, THE US SUPREME COURT affirmed that the state could not prohibit a married couple's use of contraception, because to do so would infringe on a couple's constitutionally guaranteed zone of privacy.[1] A few years later, in its Eisenstadt decision, the Court reaffirmed this view, but it also specified that this inviolable zone of privacy pertained not only to the married couple but also to each individual.[2] In both cases, the context and setting of the use of contraception were presumed to be a married couple making a rational decision about when and how often they wanted to reproduce. The earlier Griswold ruling put forth an interesting and important description of the family. Justice William O. Douglas, writing for the majority, stated that "marriage is a coming together for better or for worse, hopefully enduring, and intimate to the degree of being sacred. It is an association that promotes a way of life, not causes; a harmony in living, not political faiths; a bilateral loyalty, not commercial or social projects."[3] It is clear that for Douglas the family's domain is separate from broader political and social concerns. Family predates political institutions, and as such it must be protected from the reach of "social projects."[4]

The relationship of the individual and the family to broader social projects is the central theme of this chapter. The use of contraception as a way to respond to demographic concerns extends the scope of our discussion from sexual ethics and violence to the domain of social justice—the obligations that a society owes to all its members. This goal

130

of treating all the members of one's society justly is usually construed in Catholic parlance as the common good. In this context contraception is not merely an exercise of individual rights or of personal preference but rather is connected to a broader political and social vision. Of course, as the previous two chapters have already illustrated, individual preferences are not always easily separable from social policies. However, in this chapter we focus on a more visibly public project: population control and its relationship to a just social order. Since the early twentieth century, when anxiety about a population explosion began to escalate, the Catholic Church has consistently opposed the use of contraception and/or sterilization to respond to perceived population problems. In the contemporary period the Church is in the minority in actively discouraging artificial contraception, and also in its skepticism about the problem of overpopulation. Thus, though it allows that the use of "natural family planning" may be more acceptable, it continues to oppose all modes of artificial contraception as intrinsically evil. This opposition is not intended only to apply to personal choices made by individuals; rather, it is also to govern social policies. For this reason, the Church actively comments on and participates in the shaping of international policies regarding population. The Church acknowledges that demography is an important component of social justice and that it is worthy of sustained attention. However, its particular views about how to assess and respond to the impact of demography on the common good are much more controversial. The Church advocates for what we might call a "pronatalist" stance that encourages families to reproduce.[5] Yet it also promotes "responsible parenthood." Both these stances are framed by a particular view about the proper relationship between the family and the state.[6]

The two previous chapters addressed exceptional cases that have emerged in the years since *Humanae vitae.* One can interpret these two cases as a challenge to the Church's teaching against artificial contraception insofar as they might suggest that exceptions ought to be permitted. One can also interpret each of these cases as teaching us something more general about the morality of contraception—that it is an issue embroiled in broader debates about sexuality and violence. Thus, we saw in chapter 3 that the Church worries that by promoting condoms to stop HIV/AIDS, it will encourage and support a promiscuous sexuality. In chapter 4, the US Catholic bishops justified emergency contraceptives for rape victims as legitimate acts of "violence" against unjust aggression. But what seemed to be a simple exception was in fact complicated by other layers of violence: the rape itself, the perception that the emergency contraceptive could do violence to an embryo, and the extent to which a woman's generative process was mutilated.

In this chapter I look at what happens when contraception is framed as an issue of justice, as I trace the Vatican's views about development and population, from Pope John XXIII's 1961 encyclical letter *Mater et magistra* to recent statements issued by Pope Benedict XVI. I show that, as with the HIV/AIDS issues discussed in chapter 3, the Vatican often frames its opposition to population control measures in pragmatic terms having to do with the most effective ways to address population problems, especially as they pertain to poverty. Thus, though the moral evil of contraception remains at the heart of the Church's opposition, it is more likely to describe its opposition to artificial contraception in terms of its lack of effectiveness as a method of population control. In other words, targeting population does not adequately address the problems of society. This appeal to effectiveness leads the Vatican to frame population issues using the concepts of the Catholic tradition of social thought. Interestingly, this aligns the Vatican with disparate groups that do not share its views about contraception but would certainly agree with this approach to justice.[7]

I begin the chapter with a brief discussion of the radical changes that have occurred in the public policy conversations about the relationship of population control and economic development. This is a complex matter that at times in its history has been connected to ideas about eugenics, immigration, and the geopolitical divide between "north" and "south." I then analyze the main official Catholic documents on these issues in order to identify the various types of arguments that the Vatican uses to support a "pronatalist" stance. In addition to the official documents, the Church also engages in public debates about its position on contraception as it pertains to population control, gender, and social justice in various other forums. Two historical incidents are especially instructive. The first, which occurred almost one hundred years ago, was the heated battle between Margaret Sanger, a strong proponent of birth control, and Father John A. Ryan, a leading spokesman for and theorist of Catholic teaching about poverty and social justice. The other incident, which occurred in the 1990s, was the Church's very public attempt to change the tone and content of the United Nations' 1994 Cairo conference's positions on birth control and population. These two historical moments, separated by seven decades, point to several important insights that connect the various themes of this book. In particular, they show that, when placed in the context of poverty and social justice, the discourse about contraception is transformed. It is no longer framed by concerns about sexual immorality and violence. Rather, when beliefs about social justice and the common good provide the primary frame of reference, the discourse about contraception is embedded in other discourses about poverty, the economy, security, and peace. As was noted in chapter 1, Catholic teaching about social justice is embodied by the Seventh Commandment, "Thou shalt not steal." Placed alongside our discussion of contraception as a violation of the Sixth Commandment in chapter 3, and of contraception as a violation of the Fifth Commandment in chapter 4, this chapter fills in the missing piece that completes the range of Catholic justifications for opposing artificial contraception.

## POPULATION AND DEVELOPMENT:
## A BRIEF HISTORY

Two competing narratives—both with fairly long histories—frame modern Catholic thinking about population and contraception.[8] One narrative claims that population numbers are shrinking, especially in Europe, and that this decrease in population results partly from the greater availability of contraception. The other narrative holds that population rates are growing exponentially, and that this growth leads to poverty and misery in many parts of the world—and even worse, to potential environmental devastation.[9] The earlier narrative, especially as it relates to the modern Catholic doctrine of contraception, can be traced back to the nineteenth century, when the populations of certain European countries, particularly France, were in decline. John Noonan cites the drop in France's population as having "the greatest immediate impact on Catholic teaching," mainly because France in the nineteenth century was one of the largest Catholic countries.[10] When the French clergy began to notice the decline in births, they directed inquiries to the Vatican—inquiries that formed the basis of the Church's contemporary teaching about birth control. As Noonan describes this situation, there is little doubt that France experienced a significant decline in population in the nineteenth century. More controversial, however, is the precise cause of the decline—one that is especially remarkable in that it occurred several decades before such declines were felt in other Western European countries. Noonan rejects many of the common explanations, such as urbanization, later marriage age, a genetically linked decline in fertility, and the rise of rationalism. Instead, he asserts with some certainty that the only plausible explanation was the spread of contraception. He posits that this phenomenon was not motivated by political and social ideals but was rather a "widespread individual decision."[11] Thus, unlike "the birth control movement," which was to develop in the early twentieth century, the practices of individual French citizens were not motivated by ideological concerns about demography.

A starkly different narrative claims that population is growing at an exponential rate and that ultimately the planet will be unable to support such a large number of humans. The 1968 publication of Paul Ehrlich's *The Population Bomb* stands as an important moment in the development of this narrative.[12] A wide audience embraced his assessment that reproductive practices were leading humanity down the path to destruction. It was an audience already primed to accept the idea that a better world could only come about if the rapid growth of population could be stemmed. Ehrlich's view became the foundation of the idea that unless deliberate (and perhaps even coercive) measures were taken to slow down population growth, especially among the poor, the human race would run out of space and resources.

Today the stark images presented by Ehrlich and others like him are rejected by most individuals involved in population studies, who now recognize that there are complex and intertwined ethical and practical issues involved. Consequently, the debate about whether the population will actually "explode" has become more muted in recent years, especially as data appear to show a leveling off of the world's population.[13] Declines in population levels in developed countries lead some to express concerns about the extinction of certain peoples. Moreover, the populations of developing countries are not growing at the rate that many projected.[14] This can be attributed to various factors, including higher rates of infant mortality, greater access to health care, and economic development.

Nevertheless, concerns about overpopulation gained traction in the late 1960s and early 1970s as demographic statistics clearly showed a rapid growth in population in regions of the world beset by economic problems, and these statistics were used to project a world overrun by humans by 2150. This led to anxiety and panic about population growth and often a consequent unwillingness to recognize the complex factors that shape population growth. The massive growth in population in the early and middle twentieth century was due partly to increased access to health care, as well as public health initiatives that were able to increase life spans. However, fertility rates were also negatively affected by other social factors. These factors—ranging from urbanization to increased access to education to more freedoms for women—present a complex picture that undermines the traditional and overly simplistic overpopulation narrative. As one example, Betsy Hartmann points out how reproduction holds different meanings for various groups of people. So, whereas proponents of population control believe that having too many children causes danger to present and future generations, people living in environments of great impoverishment see children as their only hope for survival. For them, reproduction compensates for the high rates of infant mortality.[15]

According to Hartmann, Ehrlich's views were the source of what she calls "the myth of overpopulation." She describes it as follows: "More people equal fewer resources and more hunger, poverty, environmental degradation, and political instability." The danger of this myth, in her view, was that it distanced those living in affluent societies from the poor. It perpetuated the idea that the poor are responsible for their own poverty because of their unwillingness to control reproduction. Essentially, the population bomb/explosion metaphor was troubling because it oversimplified a very complex set of issues concerning population and development. The myth of overpopulation, writes Hartmann, was "based on fear, not understanding."[16]

Before Ehrlich's population explosion theory in the 1960s, ideas about overpopulation had been shaped by a range of philosophical movements. The starting point for these views is generally attributed to Thomas Malthus, the late-eighteenth/early-nineteenth-century British cleric who posed the idea that the world's population is destined to grow exponentially, and that such growth cannot be sustained by the Earth's limited resources, especially in terms of providing food. In essence, he posits that agricultural production can only grow arithmetically but that populations will increase exponentially. He has little confidence in humanity's ability to solve this problem through reasoned action; rather, he believes that the experience of extreme poverty will serve to override humans' desires to reproduce.[17] Even though his precise predictions about population have not materialized, his concerns about a population crisis and its connections to poverty continue to attract many followers, who develop these ideas in several directions. As Rao and Sexton note, however, "facts and figures have never had much effect on population debates and disagreements over policies because, deep down, the disagreements are political and economic disagreements, always tinged with an element of the cultural, not scientific ones."[18] For example, Malthusian ideas about population were widely resisted by Marxists, who were worried that reducing family size would also reduce the number of workers, and that decreasing their suffering would mean that they would no longer be taken up by the revolutionary desire to overthrow the proletariat.[19]

Other important figures in the development of ideas about population control were C. V. Drysdale and his wife Bessie Drysdale, the leaders of the British neo-Malthusian League, and Havelock Ellis, the influential sex psychologist and theorist. Both the Drysdales and Ellis played influential roles in shaping the prominent ideas about birth regulation in the early twentieth century. Their role was felt primarily through their influence on Margaret Sanger, who is considered to be the founder of the birth control movement in America and is responsible for coining the term "birth control." Sanger and others involved in the early birth control movement are often associated with the eugenics movement, which had roots in Darwinian social evolution, Malthusian beliefs, and colonialist imperialism. Francis Galton, an important pioneer in the eugenics movement, believed that humans must take control of breeding as a way to ensure a better and more prosperous world. Eugenicists embraced this idea and argued that by encouraging and rewarding the breeding of those considered superior and discouraging the breeding of those considered inferior, humanity would be improved.[20] It would make sense that there would be a connection between eugenics and the birth control movement, in that they both supported the view that human reproduction should not be left to fate. As we shall see in our discussion of Sanger, her rationalizations and motivations for preaching the message of birth control changed over time, but her early association with the eugenicists was significant for shaping her ideas as well as influencing the way others, especially Catholics, reacted to her ideas.

Ehrlich popularized the modern idea of the imminent threat posed by overpopulation, but it was an idea that had been brewing in the United States for more than a century. Unlike Malthus's concerns about inadequate resources to sustain populations, the Cold War provided a different context in the United States, whereby people became motivated by fears about large masses of "underdeveloped" people. In the late 1950s, President Dwight D. Eisenhower convened a committee chaired by William H. Draper Jr. to examine the various security threats to the United States. The committee's final report featured overpopulation as one such threat and recommended that US foreign aid "should heed requests for assistance from nations trying to curb runaway population."[21] Eisenhower distanced himself from this position, stating at a press conference that "this government will not, as long as I am here, have a positive political doctrine in its program that has to do with this problem of birth control. That's not our business."[22] By the time of Lyndon Johnson's presidency, the notion that birth control was "not our business" had been replaced by the idea that family planning was an important component of efforts to fight poverty both in the United States and abroad.[23] This linkage between family planning and poverty ensured that the issue became very much the government's business.

The broad-based governmental support of population control programs in the mid-1960s began to erode in 1973 with the US Supreme Court's *Roe v. Wade* decision, which legalized abortions in the first trimester. As Michelle Goldberg notes, *Roe v. Wade* "motivated an entirely new level of antiabortion activism." She suggests that as American antiabortion politicians felt their power receding in the United States in the immediate wake of *Roe v. Wade*, they turned more eagerly to the international scene. The most significant result was the Helms Amendment to the 1972 Foreign Assistance Act, which essentially banned the US Agency for International Development from funding abortion "as a method of family planning."[24] This amendment was the first step in a major reversal of US political opinion about international family planning. With the election of Ronald Reagan as president in 1980, the conservative prolife movement gained even more influence, which led to a complete turnaround in US policy. In contrast to the United States' position as a leader of international family planning efforts in the 1950s and 1960s, by 1984 it was officially claiming that economic reform, especially in the form of laissez-faire capitalism, was the answer to the population issue—not birth control.[25]

This new atmosphere led to the passage of what has come to be known as the global gag rule, which intensified and extended the Helms Amendment. According to this 1984 rule, the United States was not permitted to support organizations that actively performed or promoted abortion—even if those groups were using separate funds not received from the United States. And according to this rule, the promotion of abortion included referring women to abortion providers and also any public advocacy for legal changes to abortion laws. The rule came about partly as a response to the United Nations Population Planning Conference held in Mexico City in 1984.[26] The rule was rescinded less than a decade later, in 1993, by President Bill Clinton. But it was then reinstated in 2001 by President George W. Bush. President Barack Obama repealed it days after his inauguration in 2009, and he also reinstated US funding for the UN Population Fund.[27] We shall see later in this chapter how the Catholic Church has been involved in much of this history of US population policy.

The United Nations began to examine and actively pursue family planning programs in the 1950s, and UN delegates from Catholic countries were the first to oppose such programs. At the UN World Population Conference in Rome in 1954, all the delegates agreed that "cooperative action by members required respect for different ethical and religious values."[28] This attitude of respect for different ethical and religious values meant that the Catholic delegates at least had a chance to limit the UN's active involvement in population planning programs. By 1966, however, the situation had changed dramatically, as more people became convinced that population planning was the key element for resolving what was perceived as a growing crisis. The influence of Catholic voices, which had been central in earlier years, receded, and over time the Catholic view about population has become more and more marginalized, especially as the Church has continued to maintain its strong opposition to the use of artificial contraceptives. As we shall see, however, the Vatican has remained vocal and active in presenting its views at international conferences, such as the 1994 UN Cairo Conference.

The American Catholic context for thinking about population control was markedly different from the European one, where population rates after World War II were on the decline. By contrast, the war led to a significant increase in America's national birthrate, which continued to rise until it peaked in 1957, with Catholic fertility patterns exceeding those of the general population.[29] One can presume that this demographic pattern was largely the result of an increased sense of confidence that Americans felt for their future after emerging from the war as a world power.[30] Although this postwar period saw a rise in population, the war influenced popular opinions about population in a different direction. Some felt that war was caused by the struggles that arise from increases in population. In one historian's words, "the Second World War proved all too clearly the consequences of what happens when nations experience food and natural resource shortages and the lack of living space to support populations."[31] A new Malthusian-inspired attitude took hold, fueled by anxieties about the possibility that another world war might result if populations, especially those of Africa and Asia, continued to grow unchecked. Thus, concerns about population growth were often couched in the language of national security, and for Americans these concerns were diverted to paying attention to population growth on other continents. As a result, global population control came to be equated with the prevention of another world war.[32]

For American Catholics in the 1960s, competing narratives about population often led to conflicted responses. When viewed as part of US efforts to keep the world at peace, international population policies were easier to support. For many Catholics, their devotion to national interests led them to support these efforts. However, this narrative of controlling world population in order to promote peace and security conflicted with the Catholic rhetoric against artificial contraception. Yet, as we have seen, by the mid-1950s the Church had embraced natural fertility control, and by the 1960s it was touting "responsible parenthood." In addition to the global implications of population growth, a more troubling and interesting shift occurred in the 1960s, when some population control advocates in the United States turned their vision toward the social consequences of overpopulation in the United States. This raised a problem for Catholics, especially the hierarchy, which had supported Lyndon Johnson's War on Poverty. The US bishops were thus hesitant to condemn federal support for family planning programs outright.[33] They did insist, however, that federal programs should be noncoercive and that families should be informed about a wide range of family planning options, including the rhythm method.[34]

As I have noted, the Church continues to be actively involved in global policy discussions on these issues. How might we situate its position on population control and development in the context of other more commonly held secular positions? Frank Furedi's three distinct stages in the history of discussions about the role of population in development policies can help us answer this question, because they illustrate the conflicted status of the relationship of population and poverty. For the period 1940–55, Furedi claims that the process of development, understood as increased economic opportunities and an embrace of Western values, was viewed as the only way to resolve the perceived problem of rapid population growth, especially in societies in the Southern Hemisphere.[35] The prevailing attitude was that as countries developed, their rate of population growth would slow. In other words, population growth was a symptom of poverty, which meant that it could only be resolved if economic development resolved the severe poverty of many nations. In the second stage, which Furedi identifies as beginning in 1955, the relationship between development and population was completely reversed as a new theory gained ascendancy—one that claimed that population growth was an impediment to development. In this view, poverty was seen as a symptom of population growth. Furedi writes: "By the late fifties the view that overpopulation was primarily responsible for Third World poverty and for the consequent instability was widely accepted in official circles."[36] Thus, population growth had to be controlled before a country could hope to achieve comfortable levels of economic development. The third stage, which covers the period since 1975, is one where the link between population and development has decreased significantly. In this new paradigm, the concept of development is replaced by the idea of women's empowerment, especially through increased access to reproductive services. Furedi points to the 1994 Cairo Conference, which I discuss later in the chapter, as an example of the disappearance of development as a concern linked to population.

These radical changes in the way Western policy analysts have understood the relationship between population and poverty correlate with the way in which contemporary societies have responded to fears about overpopulation. In the earlier period the common view was that a lack of control of population was a symptom of underdeveloped countries. This led to a response that focused on economic development—a response that was often implicated in imperialist and colonialist projects and ideals. By the late 1950s, the view that underdevelopment was the result of overpopulation led to an emphasis on how to control population growth. Of course, this period coincided with the availability of the recently developed birth control pill, which made the prospect of fertility control on a massive scale more achievable. Finally, the most recent iteration of the development, poverty, and population triad is a complete rejection of the metaphor of development and all that it signifies. This view is premised on the idea that fertility control ought to be conceived as about one thing: women's choices about and access to a wide range of reproductive services. This most recent phase does not, in Furedi's view, capture the entire landscape of views about population and economic development. He admits that there are a wide range of positions about how best to conceive of this relationship. Among this range, he identifies "the religious pronatalist perspectives." These, he claims, are perspectives held by religious opponents to population policies, who argue on the basis of their opposition to any interference with the act of reproduction. Although this position certainly exists, we shall see in the next section that the Catholic Church combines the pronatalist perspective with a more complex set of views about development—ones that do not necessarily fit neatly into the three-stage schema proposed by Furedi.

## OFFICIAL CATHOLIC TEACHING ON POPULATION AND DEVELOPMENT

The Church's discourse about development and populations is a much richer version of what Furedi refers to as the "religious pronatalist perspective," insofar as it wants to take both economic realities and metaphysical beliefs into account. An example is seen in this passage from Pope John Paul II's letter to the secretary-general of the International Conference on Population and Development before the 1994 population and development conference in Cairo. John Paul II writes:

> True development cannot consist in the simple accumulation of wealth and in the greater availability of goods and services, but must be pursued with due consideration for the social, cultural and spiritual dimensions of the human being. Development programmes must be built on justice and equality, enabling people to live in dignity, harmony and peace. They must respect the cultural heritage of peoples and nations, and those social qualities and virtues that reflect the God-given dignity of each and every person and the divine plan which calls all persons to unity.

Importantly, men and women must be active agents of their own development, for to treat them as mere objects in some scheme or plan would be to stifle that capacity for freedom and responsibility which is fundamental to the good of the human person.[37]

One can see that though the pope supports the concept of development, he offers a vision of development that extends beyond economic policies that focus on material goods. He bases his vision of development on an intrinsic connection between spiritual well-being, morality, security, stewardship, and justice. Later in the letter, he makes clear that he opposes any framing of "population issues in terms of individual 'sexual and reproductive rights,' or even in terms of 'women's rights.'"[38] He bases this opposition on an expanded vision of development rather than an explicit opposition to contraception. This view, which is typical of Catholic discourse on this issue, cannot be adequately captured by Furedi's reductionist phrase "pronatalist perspectives."

John Paul II's vision expressed in the letter to the United Nations Population Fund (UNFPA) expressed the concept known in Catholicism as "integral development," which was most fully developed by Pope Paul VI in his 1967 encyclical letter *Populorum progressio*. For Paul VI, "integral development" acknowledges the importance of development while ensuring that it was understood as part of a more holistic and integrated ethical framework. He states: "Development cannot be limited to mere economic growth. In order to be authentic, it must be complete: integral, that is, it has to promote the good of every man and of the whole man."[39] He believes that social progress must always accompany economic progress. In his view, social progress is based on ideas about what it means to be human: "And man is only truly man in as far as, master of his own acts and judge of their worth, he is author of his own advancement, in keeping with nature which was given to him by his Creator and whose possibilities and exigencies he himself freely assumes."[40]

Both John Paul II's quotation and Paul VI's encyclical are difficult to place in Furedi's schema of three stages of thought about development and population. They clearly reject the view characteristic of the second stage that sees population control as a way to reduce poverty and encourage economic growth. The third stage, which claims women's empowerment as the central metaphor of population policy, would be problematic for them because it emphasizes unlimited procreative liberty at the expense of other values. The first (pre-1955) stage would seem to be the most appealing to both popes, yet it offers a view of development that focuses mostly on economic growth and misses the larger context. In these passages from John Paul II and Paul VI, one can see that for them, population control is not the only or central issue for development policies. Undoubtedly, their perspectives were shaped, and to some extent complicated, by their strong views about the immorality of artificial contraception.

For example, Paul VI, who a year later would issue his encyclical letter devoted to contraception (*Humanae vitae*), gives little attention to the morality of contraception in *Populorum*. He identifies the family as the central milieu in which humanity can achieve this mastery. Surprisingly, however, he does not stress the procreative role of the family but focuses instead on its natural state as monogamous and stable. He describes it as a place where individuals "help one another to grow wiser," but he also acknowledges that in the past the family's "influence may have been excessive to the detriment of the fundamental rights of the individual."[41] He follows this general discussion of the family as both a haven and as potentially oppressive immediately with his discussion of population—to which he refers as "accelerated demographic increase."[42] The reader is left to presume that there is a connection between the two, although the pope does not draw the connection explicitly.

One can imagine that at the time that Paul VI issued *Populorum*, many were eager to learn whether he intended to revise the Church's teaching on artificial contraception. They might have hoped that his discussion of population planning in this encyclical would offer clues, but there are very few. Paul VI acknowledges that population growth could possibly outstrip the availability of resources and that public authorities "can intervene, within the limit of their competence." Yet he never specifies what those interventions might be, describing them merely in terms of "appropriate information" and "suitable measures." He clarifies this point by indicating that these interventions must meet two requirements: They must be in conformity with the moral law, and they must respect married couples' freedom to decide the size of their families. He also addresses married couples in this passage, urging them to follow their consciences in making such decisions. He reminds them that a proper conscience is one "enlightened by God's law authentically interpreted."[43] As this brief passage makes evident, the pope never directly describes the Church's position on artificial contraception. His concerns about development and population are framed in terms of protecting the family from undue interference from the state and encouraging individuals to follow the moral law guided by their conscience. The only mention of artificial contraception is indirect; in a footnote, he points to relevant passages from the Vatican II document *Gaudium et spes*—passages that, as we saw in chapter 2, were themselves rather indefinite.[44]

To fully understand the ideal of integral development, we must backtrack historically to the writings of Pope John XXIII, especially his encyclical letter *Mater et magistra* (*On Recent Development of the Social Question in the Light of the Christian Teaching*), which was written six years before Paul VI's *Populorum*. John XXIII emphasizes that if economic growth is not accompanied by "a corresponding social development," it will fail in achieving social justice.[45] He devotes much of the letter to outlining the important recent changes in economic arrangements, as well as the conditions and contexts of work. He also attends to claims that population growth is increasing at such a rapid rate that the world's inhabitants will soon outstrip its available economic resources. In particular, he addresses the idea that the only solution to this potential dilemma would be to limit procreation. His response is framed by skepticism about the accuracy of claims about overpopulation. Nevertheless, he suggests that even if these claims were to materialize, God has "provided nature with almost inexhaustible productive capacity" and humans "with such ingenuity that, by using suitable means, [they] can apply nature's resources to the needs and requirements of existence."[46] He is firm in his insistence that it is unacceptable to respond to the pressures of population growth by acting "contrary to the moral law laid down by God." More directly, he asserts that the "procreative function" cannot be violated.[47]

John XXIII saw contraception as immoral because he believed that it went against God's inviolate law—a law that protects the sanctity of human life and affirms God's role as creator of life. He appealed broadly to natural law and its emphasis on "the plan of God," which suggested that means of limiting births are "contrary to human reason."[48] He was confident that humans would be able to rely on their ingenuity to ensure that sufficient resources are available to all humans. Yet he also acknowledged that though there were burdens associated with the procreation of children, these burdens must be met with dignity and are never a sufficient cause for violating God's laws.

Both John Paul II (in 1987) and Benedict XVI (in 2009) commemorated Paul VI's encyclical letter *Populorum progressio*. In their commemorations, they reiterated and confirmed their predecessor's views but also expanded on them to reflect contemporary concerns. They confronted the issue of population and development, an important aspect of Paul VI's document, but in a way that reflected the changes that had occurred in the intervening decades. In *Solicitudo rei socialis*, marking the twentieth anniversary of *Populorum*, John Paul II addresses the issue of population as it is related to development. He uses the term "demographic problem" to capture the idea that not only overpopulation in certain regions but also a drop in the birthrate in other regions are concerns. He points out that population decreases can also hinder development and that the notion that "*all* demographic growth is incompatible with orderly development" has not been proven.[49] Nevertheless, most of his comments address attempts by certain countries to institute national birth control campaigns. This type of coercion is, in his view, the ultimate threat to true and authentic human development. He does not present the moral justifications for the Church's stance against contraception, but he uses the opportunity to frame birth control campaigns as violations of respect for individual freedom. He calls this a "new form of oppression" that ultimately runs the risk of embracing racist ideologies that could lead to forms of eugenics.[50] John Paul II also condemns this type of birth control by linking it with a type of cultural hegemony, where "pressure and financing coming from abroad" work to undermine the religious and cultural identities of certain developing countries.[51] In particular, he identifies policies where financial aid is given to developing countries on the condition that they will provide reproductive services.

John Paul II's encyclical letter reframes the issue of population control in two significant ways. First, he expands it beyond overpopulation to also address the problem of demographic decline. Second, he grounds opposition to birth control in a notion of reproductive freedom—a term usually associated with the birth control movement. The pope strengthens this move by invoking the specter of eugenics. Although he does not use the term in this document, his view is part of what he refers to in an earlier encyclical letter as an "anti-life mentality."[52] For John Paul II, this term describes what occurs when humans, who are overcome by fear and anxiety about the future of the human

race, fail to have faith and confidence in God. Worries about overpopulation are, in his view, an example of this unbridled anxiety: "One
thinks, for example, of a certain panic deriving from the studies of ecol-
ogists and futurologists on population growth, which sometimes exag-
gerate the danger of demographic increase to the quality of life." Only
a paragraph later, however, the pope acknowledges "the serious problem
of population growth," but he deems the moral implication of this
growth to be that the Church must confirm even more strongly its
teaching on contraception.[53]

Pope Benedict XVI chose the theme of "integral development" as
the centerpiece of his first encyclical on social thought. He expresses
his belief that Pope Paul VI's teachings warrant revisiting in terms of
new developments in society. In the encyclical, Benedict emphasizes
the following points. First, he situates *Populorum* in the context of
Paul's other encyclicals, especially *Humanae vitae*. He argues that the
teachings of *Humanae* are not purely a matter of individual morality but
rather that they reveal the strong link between "life ethics and social
ethics."[54] In particular, he identifies the contradiction he sees in societies that claim to value human dignity and human rights yet also support what he views as antilife actions. It is clear in this document that
for Benedict, the primary evil of contraception is that it devalues life.
Yet he also gestures toward the social justice implications of decisions
about human life.

Mostly, however, the purpose of Benedict's encyclical is to show how
the context of development has changed in the period since *Populorum*.
He identifies in great detail all the changes that have occurred, including changes in how society views contraception. He frames the morality
of contraception as a matter of respect for and acceptance of life, and
he reiterates many of John Paul II's ideas about an antibirth mentality
that has taken hold of developed countries and is being exported to
underdeveloped countries under the guise of cultural progress.[55] More
than his predecessors, Benedict offers an explicit account of the connection between a prolife (or acceptance-for-life) mentality and economic
development. Essentially, he claims that when people are open to life,
three things follow. First, there is an increase in empathy, whereby
wealthy people can better understand the needs of the poor. Second,
openness to life leads citizens to better utilize resources by avoiding
using them merely to pursue selfish desires. Third, this attitude toward
life promotes virtuous action by contributing to the moral growth and

development of citizens.[56] This encyclical illustrates Benedict's ability to transform an anticontraception stance into a pro–human rights stance that expresses solidarity with the poor. Essentially, he says that a rejection of artificial contraception is a more effective way to bring about social change. He appeals to the consequences of this position as good reasons to embrace the Catholic opposition to contraception. This justificatory move is familiar to us, for we have seen it in the discussion about condoms and HIV/AIDS. In both cases the Church replaces a focus on sex and harm—the two primary categories it uses to evaluate contraception—with a focus on social justice. And in both cases, effectiveness is invoked as a way to counteract those who argue that contraceptives are effective solutions, both to the HIV/AIDS epidemic and to the issue of development and population.

Benedict also introduces a profoundly theological component in his evaluation of the concept of development. He claims that those sociologists and political scientists who normally utilize the concept of development are limited by history and culture—the matters of this world. What they are actually referring to when they invoke development may more properly be referred to as growth or evolution. Their view lacks a transcendent dimension—a belief that humans "possess a nature destined to transcend itself in a supernatural life."[57] Without such a dimension, true, integral development is not possible. In the context of a secular framework, humanity can grow and evolve—but that is different from development. Development properly entails a view to the transcendent. It is also a teleological concept insofar as it entails a proper perfection of a thing's nature. This appeal to theology correlates with earlier discussions of development as the integration of the material and spiritual. To a certain extent, this type of appeal undermines the relatability of the Church's position, and for this reason the Church also appeals to pragmatic and prudential supports for its position.

The journey from John XXIII's early ideas about population and development to Benedict XVI's teachings was marked by fundamental change as well as by some consistency. One noteworthy change is that unlike John XXIII, Benedict is relatively silent about whether or not population growth is of serious concern. Moreover, Benedict's explanation of the link between contraception and social justice is more theological and optimistic, insofar as it notes the positive benefits of natural family planning. These various statements also represent a remarkable consistency. While responding to the realities and popular theories of their times, they never waver from their belief in the unchanging and absolute nature of the Church's teaching on contraception.

## POVERTY, POPULATION, AND JUSTICE: MARGARET SANGER AND JOHN A. RYAN

Official Vatican statements can be insular; they are not an invitation to dialogue and debate. There are times, however, when the Church engages directly in dialogue and public policy negotiations with non-Catholics on the issue of contraception. We turn to two examples, both from the American context, to examine the implications of such negotiations, especially how they clarify the category of justice in Catholic views on contraception. The first example is the public debate in the 1930s between the birth control activist Margaret Sanger and Father John A. Ryan, a spokesman for Catholic social justice. The second is the Vatican's aggressive intervention in the UNFPA's Cairo Conference in 1994.

Sanger played a significant role in making birth control a central feature of American sexual practice. Various chapters of the story of her crusade to make birth control widely available involve the American Catholic Church, mainly through Sanger's engagement with various clerics, including Ryan. Ryan was the influential Catholic social activist best known for his advocacy of the just living wage. As head of the Social Action Department of the National Catholic Welfare League in the early twentieth century, Ryan helped to shape the teachings of the US Catholic bishops on issues related to social welfare and justice.[58] The contrast between Sanger's and Ryan's views is significant because it highlights several important features of the morality of contraception, especially as they pertain to the argument of this book. First, both Sanger and Ryan were deeply concerned about poverty and social justice, and yet they came to two very different conclusions about the importance of population planning. Second, both their views were shaped in very different ways by eugenics. Sanger embraced the concept early in her career and then later distanced herself from it. Ryan viewed eugenics as a dangerous policy that unfairly attacked the poor and violated Catholic teachings on contraception. Third, their radically different views about sexual morality shaped their attitudes about the morality of contraception. Sanger believed that birth control would improve sexual relations between men and women. It would free the world from "sexual prejudice and taboo, by demanding the frankest and most unflinching reexamination of sex in its relation to human nature and the bases of society."[59] By contrast, Ryan held that people's desires to use birth control were motivated by material pleasure at the expense of morality.

Much of the writing about Sanger's life is highly polemical.[60] There is no doubt that she was an incendiary figure in her day; her tactics were aggressive, and she associated with prominent radicals. She and her husband were arrested in the United States for violating the Comstock Laws—which made advertisements or any printed matter about contraception illegal to disperse through the US mail—by speaking publicly about contraception and distributing information about it, but by the end of her life, the US government shared her views about birth control. In 1963, President John F. Kennedy offered tentative support for contraceptive research, and within five years, the government fully supported and embraced the link between contraception and population control. In his State of the Union Address in 1965, President Lyndon Johnson pledged to "seek new ways to use our knowledge to help deal with the explosion in world population and the growing scarcity of world resources."[61] This shift in the conversation about birth control from the realm of personal morality to the public sphere was brought about largely by Sanger's efforts. She spoke publicly about the issue, and she insisted that birth control was tied to a range of social, economic, and political issues. The historical assessments of her life are mixed, partly because of her personal choices about family life, but mostly because of her strong association with and endorsement of the eugenics movement. Thus she often poses a difficult problem for feminist scholars, who appreciate her contribution to promoting freedom for women but are troubled by her embrace of racial eugenic philosophies.[62]

Although Sanger began her career advocating birth control as a way to help poor women, she shifted her emphasis later in her career as she embraced certain tenets of the eugenics movement. Instead of viewing poor women as victims, she came to view them and their high birthrates as a problem that was harmful to society. The history of her views is instructive insofar as it shows how difficult it is to separate concerns about class, race, and gender from discussions about contraception. Some have attributed these shifts in her views to her ambition and single-minded desire to make easy and safe contraception available to all women. Essentially, she used four types of justifications to support her views about the positive impact of birth control: (1) Contraception enhances women's sexual experiences, (2) contraception improves women's health and well-being, (3) contraception helps to stabilize population growth, and (4) contraception can advance eugenics goals. Throughout her career Sanger shifted between these various arguments—a quality that some biographers have depicted negatively.[63]

Sanger engaged in the fight for access to birth control on several fronts. She supported making contraception a part of medical practice, and to that end she fought to ensure that laws were passed to limit dispensing contraception to physicians. Physicians had been reluctant to embrace contraception. They worried about its association with "lay medicine," its use for purposes that were not pathological, and the lack of rigorous testing about its successes and failures.[64] She also pursued safer and more effective modes of contraception. She played an important role in funding the scientific research that was the basis for the development of the hormonal contraceptive pill in the 1950s.[65] On the legal and legislative fronts, she fought to overturn both those laws that made contraception illegal and the Comstock Laws.[66]

Sanger went to great lengths to target the Catholic Church as the primary obstacle to efforts to change attitudes about fertility and reproduction. Many scholars have interpreted Sanger's attitudes toward Catholicism as a virulent anti-Catholicism that stemmed from her father's distinct hatred of his own Catholicism. Kennedy concludes from her personal papers that her "childhood obsession with supposed Catholic deviousness" became more and more exaggerated as she grew older.[67] Although Kennedy's overly psychological assessment of Sanger's attitudes toward the Church might be difficult to prove, some of her own writing exhibits the strength of her negative feelings about the Church. For example, she attributed nefarious motives to the Church's opposition to birth control—such as, for example, fear of allowing women too much freedom and the need for "a high birthrate to provide laymen to support its increasingly expensive organization."[68] The US Catholic establishment reacted forcefully to Sanger and her views. Yet, as Kennedy notes, "Each side had to share the blame for the degradation of the dialogue on birth control."[69] Though Ryan and other Catholic clerics engaged in less sophisticated debates with Sanger, in his own writing, Ryan offered a careful and reasoned response to her specific attempts to present birth control as a remedy for poverty. As was noted above, Ryan, like Sanger, was a strong advocate on behalf of the poor.

Ryan is best known for his role in the development of economic policies, particularly his advocacy for the living wage. His support of the New Deal was influential in shaping US public policy in the pre–World War II period. Yet in his role as adviser to the Catholic National Welfare Conference, he was called upon to respond to claims that birth control initiatives were an effective way to address the growing problem of poverty. In testifying before the US Senate in 1934, he clearly explained that claims that contraception would better the lot of the poor "divert the attention of influential classes from the pursuit of social justice and to relieve them of all responsibility for our bad distribution and other social maladjustments."[70] In essence, he was expressing a concern that has come to characterize much contemporary thinking about family planning and overpopulation: that a singular emphasis on population control somehow places the blame on the poor themselves and makes them responsible for their misery. For Ryan, the issue of family limitation was part of larger social and economic concerns. His view predates the concept of integral development described in the papal statements that were discussed earlier in this chapter, but his emphasis on placing population concerns in as broad a context as possible is very similar. In the US Catholic bishops' 1919 pastoral letter issued by James Cardinal Gibbons, which Ryan was said to have helped draft, we read that though individuals are driven to limit the size of their families either for selfish reasons or because they believe that it will help the species, eventually it is the nation that will suffer: "The harm which it does cannot be repaired by social service, nor offset by pretended economic or domestic advantage."[71]

Ryan explains the Catholic position against contraception in more detail in a brochure titled "Family Limitation and the Church and Birth Control." His description of the Catholic view is especially pertinent to this chapter because it addresses the various modes of argument utilized to defend birth control. He began by asserting that the terms "birth control," "birth restriction," "contraceptives," and "contraception" have all been devised as part of a deliberate attempt "to make known and recommend to the poorer classes devices for the limitation of their families."[72] He wants to help Catholics understand the basis of the Church's opposition, which he describes as primarily metaphysical, and then to respond to the social utility argument relied on by opponents of the

Church. He is also concerned that certain Catholics have convinced themselves that the Church's teaching about the use of contraceptive devices allows for occasional exceptions. He believes that the Church offers rational and intelligible reasons for opposing all "positive methods of birth prevention," including abortion.

His explication of the Catholic teaching is strongly grounded in Thomistic natural law; he discusses the natural ends of faculties and asserts that any use of a human faculty for an unnatural end is wrong. In the context of sex, the natural purpose of the sexual organs is procreation; thus, deliberately blocking that purpose would be sinful. He adds that there is no exception to this rule. For him, this moral justification coheres with his Catholic worldview that bases moral evaluations on the demands of natural law. However, he acknowledges that this metaphysical framework will not appeal to all persons, especially those who rely on the model of social utility, a view that he believes is similarly grounded in metaphysical assumptions. He describes the utilitarian as follows: "He must assume that social utility is good in itself, intrinsically good. Thus, his fundamental position took the form of a metaphysical principle." He adds, "In this respect we are on equal footing."[73] He distinguishes natural law from social utility models in several ways, but one distinction is notable. He claims that the natural law argument appeals to the intellect—the mind of the believer. But he acknowledges how much more appealing the concept of social utility is to the lived experiences of believers, mainly because of its emotional appeal to notions like neighborly love and avoiding harm.

On the basis of his belief that utilitarian arguments have more traction with the populace, Ryan presents several such arguments in defense of the Catholic opposition to contraception. First, he argues that the use of contraceptive devices devalues marriage and leads to severe losses of faith, trust, and reverence in marriage. Second, he identifies the broader damage that occurs to the "race." He writes that a deliberate attempt to limit family size "leads inevitably to an increase of softness, luxury and materialism, and to a decrease of mental and moral discipline, of endurance, and of the power of achievements."[74] When people attempt to control family size, they tend to reject the Christian ethic that stresses sacrifice, struggle, and suffering because, in Ryan's view, such people are only motivated by "the indefinite increase and variation of pleasant physical sensations." Individuals would thus be focused on the physical and material at the expense of their moral growth and development. As a result of this kind of materialism, their service to and love of neighbor will no longer be disinterested.

A third negative consequence of limiting family size, according to Ryan, is that children raised in small families are more likely to be selfish and overly dependent on others. He admits that it might be hard to provide definite empirical evidence to support this contention. Nevertheless, he believes it to be self-evident that parents who use artificial contraceptives are taking the easy way out, and in so doing they are teaching their children a lesson that rejects the Catholic emphasis on struggle and suffering. He notes that, by contrast, couples who limit their family size using sexual abstinence are teaching their children something important about suffering and struggle. He makes an interesting point that reveals his concern that it is primarily the middle and upper classes that have embraced family-planning techniques. He acknowledges that he is not encouraging more suffering for working-class and poor families, but he worries that even if a smaller family size would get them out of poverty, they would still be harming the larger society by decreasing the general population.

Therefore, not only would the quality of humankind suffer, but so also would its quantity. Ryan was responding to a widely held belief of the time that populations were diminishing in Europe and to some extent in America. Unlike the population control movement of the 1960s, which was spurred by serious concerns about overpopulation of the planet, Ryan's context was shaped by evidence that the populations in predominantly Catholic countries were falling, a point discussed earlier in this chapter. Here, as with the previous consequence, Ryan acknowledges that the poor might benefit economically from depopulation, because fewer laborers might lead to increases in their wages, but he worries that they will become egotistical and materialistic as a result. Moreover, he asserts the view that the ends never justify the means—especially if those means are intrinsically evil.

The most passionate sections of Ryan's discussion of family limitation are his analyses of its relation to poverty. He responds to the claim that one positive consequence of family planning might be a betterment of conditions for the poor by saying that we ought to focus on a more just distribution of goods. He is concerned that those—the rich—who suggest family limitation as a remedy for poverty are simply avoiding responsibility for the working class "by showing that . . . the working poor . . . had chiefly themselves to blame."[75] He also rejects Malthus's view, basically arguing that his predictions about the lack of food were false. Improved methods of production ensured that there would be plenty of food, but he also acknowledges that a time could come when resources might be depleted; and if so, he writes that "perhaps large numbers of persons will someday be obliged to choose between temporary or permanent celibacy and long periods of abstinence within the marital union." Nevertheless, he expresses the feeling that there is no need to worry now: "Sensible persons will not cross the bridge of overpopulation until they come to it."[76]

Ryan also responded to the claims of the eugenicists and roundly rejected their views on several fronts. He is hesitant to place any impediments to marriage on entire groups of people, especially because he believes that the scientific evidence about heredity is so uncertain. Mostly, however, his response to eugenics is framed in terms of social justice, especially a living family wage. If society required employers to pay their workers sufficiently, then there would be no need for workers to limit the size of their families. Of course, Ryan thinks that the real reason that married couples are turning to contraceptives is not economic but sensual. This is supported by his belief that the majority of persons using these illicit means are from the wealthier classes. Thus, he writes: "The plain truth is that the evil is fundamentally moral rather than economic. It has its roots in a wrong view of life, and of what constitutes a worthy and reasonable life."[77]

Leslie Tentler claims that Ryan was able to maintain a complex attitude toward contraception because of some distinctively Catholic views; Catholics who embraced the belief that humans were social were suspicious of individual autonomy. It was precisely this belief that led Catholics to support the idea of the welfare state and to embrace the notion of solidarity with those who are less fortunate. Thus, in Tentler's view, Ryan's worry about contraception was that it would erode the social fiber by breaking down the family, and it would lead to a "crass materialism." His view of the person as social also led him to worry that society, by advocating contraception as a solution for poverty and misery, was eschewing its duty to care for low-wage workers and the poor. "Catholic teaching on contraception was thus for men like Ryan intimately related to a range of social welfare and social justice concerns," writes Tentler.[78] However, she does not want to discount something else at work in Ryan's view—what she calls "a celibate's understanding of marital sex, tinctured with a strong dose of Victorian prudery."[79] This view echoes Sanger's suspicion about the real motivations for the

Catholic views against contraception. We see once again how the target of contraception—be it sexual immorality, harm, or justice—is continually moving.

Although Sanger and Ryan shared a desire to help improve living conditions for the poor, they diverged on how birth control could be used to achieve that goal. Sanger saw birth control as a potential savior for the poor, especially women; but for Ryan, contraception was ultimately a violation of God's law that would also lead to negative consequences for society. He believed that poverty could be addressed through economic reforms and could thus be alleviated without requiring families to limit their size. Both Sanger and Ryan were motivated by a sense of justice; both wanted humans to flourish, and both believed that communities had a responsibility to support that flourishing. Yet they had radically different visions of what that flourishing entailed and how to achieve it. Ryan's insistence on social justice and his rejection of eugenics certainly puts him on the right side of history, especially in light of the horrors perpetrated in the twentieth century in the name of eugenics. Sanger, in spite of her embrace of eugenics, fought to make sure that the issue of family planning was connected to women's emancipation and well-being—a point supported by contemporary feminist views. Ryan's patriarchal framework occluded his ability to make such a connection. In the next section we explore an example of a direct interaction between Catholic views and feminist views.

## THE CAIRO CONFERENCE, THE CATHOLIC CHURCH, AND FEMINISM

Almost seventy years since the days of Margaret Sanger and Father John Ryan, the realities of the economy, population, and development have changed drastically. Yet the divergence on what constitutes human flourishing that characterized the divide between Sanger and Ryan still persists. It can be seen more recently in the ongoing political battles between the Vatican and the population control establishment. By the 1960s and 1970s, the Catholic Church had become a significant player in the international scene. As early as the late 1950s, the US Catholic bishops had publicly opposed any US policy that linked foreign aid to population control programs. Under President Eisenhower, the Draper

Commission had stressed the importance of population control programs in nations where poverty was prevalent. This connection between foreign policy and population control shaped and defined the national view of population control. By the 1960s, the movement begun by Sanger had taken on two very distinct domains. As far as the sphere of the family was concerned, the repeal of the final Comstock Laws in Connecticut and Massachusetts ensured the removal of any obstacles to obtaining contraception and information about contraception.[80] Moreover, the widely available birth control pill made it even easier for women to regulate their reproductive cycles and avoid pregnancy. With regard to public policy, the primary concerns had to do with public funding of family planning programs, and over time the focus came to be more and more on the international funding of programs. The issue of public funding overshadowed any other debates about the ethics of contraception in the latter part of the twentieth century.

Population control is not merely a governmental enterprise. A wide range of governmental and nongovernmental agencies, groups, and individuals are involved in the delivery of family planning and reproductive services. Many of these agencies share a similar set of beliefs about family planning, women's well-being, and the common good. In 2008, the UN reported that the United States was the largest country making donations to family planning programs, donating 50 percent of all funds.[81] The major US agency involved in population planning activities is the US Agency for International Development. In addition to other developed nations, much of the funding and activity comes from the United Nations through the UNFPA, the World Bank, the International Planned Parenthood Federation, the Population Council, and the Bill & Melinda Gates, Ford, Mellon, and Rockefeller foundations.[82] The Catholic Church has fought actively against these population planning agencies since the 1960s. The battles have been both private and public, and have covered a range of contexts and issues. The most public and epic of these battles occurred in the wake of the 1994 UNFPA conference in Cairo. Under the leadership of Pope John Paul II, the Catholic Church joined forces with some unlikely allies to fight against the vision of development and family planning being proposed at the Cairo conference.

The UNFPA convened the International Conference on Population and Development in Cairo in 1994 to address the relationship between development and population—a relationship with a complex history mired in competing political and economic agendas. In a letter to the executive director of the UNFPA, Pope John Paul II urged the UNFPA and the participants in the conference to remember that "none of the issues to be discussed is simply an economic or demographic concern, but, at root, each is a matter of profound significance, with far-reaching implications."[83] The pope distilled this significance to four "basic truths": the dignity and worth of each person, human life is sacred from conception to natural death, human rights are innate and transcend any constitutional order, and the human race must strive to build a just society to promote and protect the common good.[84] His basic premise was that a development approach cannot reduce population issues to matters of individual rights but must always view them in the context of basic objective ethical truths. Although the pope clearly stated the Church's opposition to artificial contraception, his concerns in this letter were more wide-ranging. He was worried about coercive measures such as forced sterilization, and even more troubling for him was the inclusion of abortion as a tool for population control. He framed these issues in the context of a concern for families, and more particularly for children and women.

The outcome of the Cairo conference, as articulated in its twenty-year Program of Action (POA), also exhibited a concern for women, but a concern that related to women's ability to make informed and autonomous decisions about reproductive choices. Most of John Paul II's other concerns were not addressed by the POA. An excerpt from the POA's definition of reproductive health reflects the intense divide between the UN conference and the Vatican:

> Reproductive health is a state of complete physical, mental and social well-being in all matters relating to the reproductive system and to its functions and processes. It implies that people have the capability to reproduce and the freedom to decide if, when and how often to do so. Implicit in this is the right of men and women to be informed and to have access to safe, effective, affordable and acceptable methods of family planning of their choice, as well as other methods of their choice for regulation of fertility, which are not against the law, and the right of access to health-care services that will enable women to go safely through pregnancy and childbirth.[85]

One would be hard-pressed to find two such different attitudes toward reproduction as the ones represented by the Vatican and the UN. Nevertheless, one premise of this chapter is that the Catholic Church's

long-standing interest in issues related to social justice has led its representatives to deploy a wide range of justifications and moral arguments
to ground their views. It is precisely this variety that enables us to navigate between these disparate positions and to render them coherent
with each other.

The 1994 Cairo conference's shift toward a view of family planning
as an issue of human rights for women brings its position much closer
to Sanger's ideas about birth control as a way to emancipate women.
John Paul II upholds the Catholic opposition to artificial contraception,
but he connects it to a wider set of societal ills that conspire to devalue
life. Although in many ways he articulates a vision of social justice very
much in line with Ryan's, his concern with assaults on the sanctity of
life serves to make the issue of contraception primarily a matter of life
and death, rather than a matter of social justice. Moreover, in addressing the Cairo conference, the pope departed from his more typical view
of connecting contraception to sexual immorality. This is especially
interesting because he had devoted much of his papacy to advancing a
theology that framed human experience primarily through the lenses of
sexuality and gender. Nevertheless, like Ryan, the pope rejected a view
of humanity that is based on individual autonomy—a view that the
conservative Catholic commentator George Weigel claims was the core
philosophical concept at the heart of the Cairo conference's vision.[86]

The Cairo conference was the third UN conference to address the
issue of population and development.[87] By all accounts, the Cairo conference's emphasis on women's health issues came about as a result of
deliberate planning by women's rights activists who were concerned
about the lack of attention given to women's health and also by the
abuses that had taken place internationally in the name of population
control. Essentially, they wanted to ensure that women's reproductive
rights were protected, and this included both access to and information
about birth control and abortion. These activists were able to forge a
consensus with disparate groups, including influential population control advocates. One scholar suggests that population control advocates
were willing to change their approach to fertility reduction because they
realized that empowering women to make decisions about their reproduction would help them achieve their goal more efficiently.[88]

The "Cairo Consensus" has come to be associated with a major shift
in the rhetoric of population planning—a shift that is usually attributed

to the influence of feminist activists who wanted to address the concerns and needs of women globally. In particular, they succeeded in cementing the idea that information about and access to contraception is an important element of women's overall health. The conference promoted the view that women's health was critical to development. Thus, contraceptives and access to abortion were not framed as ways to control population but rather ways to empower women. Of course, the ultimate objective was that empowered women would be free to make "good" reproductive choices, which would ultimately be good for economic development.

The master plans consented to by the conference explain these connections in more detail. First, they affirm the central connection between development and population by noting that population growth both influences and is influenced by poverty and structures of social and gender inequity. The plans also assert that development strategies must integrate environmental concerns because of the important link between population, consumption, the use of natural resources, and environmental degradation. The Vatican embraced and supported this framing vision of social and environmental justice, but opposed the way the plans emphasized reproductive freedom as a central way to achieve this justice. More specifically, the document asserts that with poverty come certain challenges, including limited access to reproductive health services such as family planning. Unlike earlier approaches to population matters, these plans describe a complex relationship between poverty and population. They do not make the claim that population control will eradicate poverty. Rather, they assert that "sustained economic growth" will eradicate poverty, and the "eradication of poverty will contribute to slowing population growth."[89]

On the specific issue of family planning, the document makes some important claims. It firmly rejects any coercive population policies, arguing instead that the minimal responsibility of governments is to ensure access to information and services. The plans also urge governmental leaders to go beyond that responsibility by promoting and legitimizing reproductive control. At several points in the document, the authors stress the importance of making reproductive health services "acceptable." Nevertheless, the plans clearly emphasize that family planning is ultimately a matter of individual choice, because access to these services is primary a matter of health: "Family-planning programmes work best when they are part of or linked to broader reproductive health programmes that address closely related health needs and when women are fully involved in the design, provision, management and evaluation of services."[90]

Much of the media attention around the conference focused on the issue of abortion. The Vatican and its allies were concerned that one of the goals of the conference was to endorse the view that abortion ought to be viewed as a right to which women are entitled. More particularly, the concern was that it would be framed as a health care right. The Church and its allies were able to influence the drafting of the final report such that the language about abortion rights was toned down. Nevertheless, as the Vatican's official response to the master plans stated, "The final document, as opposed to the earlier documents of the Bucharest and Mexico City conferences, recognizes abortion as a dimension of population policy and, indeed of primary health care, even though it does stress that abortion should not be promoted as a means to family planning and urges nations to find alternatives to abortion."[91]

Pope John Paul II wrote a public letter to the conference's secretary-general objecting to the conclusions it reached. In language more pointed than the Vatican objections appended to the POA, the pope described the Catholic opposition to abortion and birth control. He also expressed his concerns about social justice. These concerns, however, were overshadowed by his insistence on metaphysical justifications—that "the Church stands opposed to the imposition of limits on family size, and to the promotion of methods of limiting births which separate the unitive and procreative dimensions of marital intercourse, which are contrary to the moral law inscribed on the human heart, or which constitute an assault on the sacredness of life."[92]

In the almost twenty years since the Cairo conference, there have been a variety of reactions to its conclusions. One type is to lament how slow governments have been to implement its POA. Others have noted that the situation of women's health worldwide has deteriorated substantially since 1994. Yet others continue to be suspicious of the conference as a hegemonic attempt by white Northern feminists to impose their worldview on other women. What has changed rather dramatically since the conference is the growing chorus of criticism toward population policies in general. The notion that there is a demographic fix has been discounted by most. Moreover, many hold that in spite of its talk of women's emancipation and reproductive rights, the Cairo conference was still beholden to a neo-Malthusian philosophy that holds a simplistic view of the relationship between population and justice more generally. Thus, just as with the public debate between Sanger and Ryan, the debate between the Vatican and the UN on these issues is complex. The complexity is due in part to the conflicting views about social justice, especially about how and whether reproductive freedoms advance justice. In other words, the Vatican and the UN hold substantially different views about what is at stake in the activity of artificial reproduction.

## CONCLUSION

This discussion of contraception as it relates to population policies helps to expand the scope of our thinking about the morality of contraception. In particular, it is a reminder that contraception is not just a private matter related to the Sixth Commandment but is just as much an issue of social justice related to the Seventh Commandment. The Catholic Church's absolute opposition to artificial contraception means that regardless of its view about the importance of the relationship of demographics and social justice, it can never accept the use of illicit means. Its embrace of natural family planning, however, does allow it to advocate for responsible parenthood—and this language of responsibility becomes a way for official teaching to incorporate ideas about the common good. Part of the problem is whether decisions that couples make about the size of their families ought to be based merely on private concerns or whether a couple can take a broader view of population and make decisions based on the common good. This is where the Catholic rhetoric on this issue is complicated, especially in the recent turn under John Paul II's and Benedict's papacies toward a rejection of the overpopulation thesis. By instead embracing the belief that populations are diminishing, or that population growth has stabilized, they reinforce the Catholic idea that the common good might actively be enhanced by increases in populations and that therefore procreation ought to be encouraged.

## NOTES

1. *Griswold v. Connecticut*, 381 US 479 (1965).
2. *Eisenstadt v. Baird*, 405 US 438 (1972).

3. *Griswold v. Connecticut* (J. Douglas, opinion of the court).

4. For an excellent study of Catholic teachings about the role of the family in society, see Cahill, *Family*.

5. The strong emphasis on reproduction has diminished in the past decades. Nineteenth- and early-twentieth-century official documents explicitly encouraged Catholics to have large families. See especially Pope Leo XIII, *Arcanum divinae sapientia* (*On Christian Marriage*).

6. There are numerous examples in Catholic social teaching of this type of discussion of the family. See, e.g., Pope Leo XII, *Rerum novarum* (*On the Condition of Labor*), par. 9–10; and Second Vatican Council, *Gaudium et spes* (*The Church in the Modern World*) (1965), par. 52.

7. An interesting case was the alliance forged between feminists and the Catholic hierarchy in Peru to oppose President Alberto Fujimoro's coercive sterilization programs in the late 1990s. See Ewig, "Hijacking Global Feminism."

8. The narrative of falling birthrates has a long history as Noonan illustrates through the first-century legislation (*Lex Julia et Papia*) designed to stimulate births among the upper classes. Noonan, *Contraception*, 20–21.

9. The narrative that links the use of contraceptives to population decline led to the passage of a law in France in the 1920s outlawing the sale of contraceptives; St. John-Stevas, *Agonising Choice*, 449.

10. Noonan, *Contraception*, 387.

11. Ibid., 394.

12. Ehrlich, *Population Bomb*.

13. In October 2012, the world celebrated the birth of its 7 billionth baby. Obviously, this was a symbolic gesture, but one that received much media coverage. See, e.g., Gomez and Sullivan, "'7 Billionth' Babies Feted."

14. The average annual rate of population growth worldwide peaked from 1965 to 1970, at 2.069 percent. The estimated rate for 2010 was 1.162 percent. Numerous European countries show negative population growth rates in 2010. United Nations, *World Population Prospects*.

15. Hartmann, *Reproductive Rights and Wrongs*, 11.

16. Ibid., 4.

17. Malthus, *Essay*.

18. Rao and Sexton, "Introduction," 6.

19. Kennedy, *Birth Control*, 75.

20. Decter, "Nine Lives," 2–3.

21. *Time*, December 14, 1959.

22. Ibid.

23. An important piece of this history is the involvement of figures like the Rockefellers and Hugh Moor in the development of Planned Parenthood, a group that has influenced much of US policy on population control. See Goldberg, *Means of Reproduction*, 37–68.

24. Ibid., 65.

25. Ibid.

26. Ibid., 99.

27. *New York Times*, "World of Harm."

28. Murphy, "Catholic Perspectives," 14.

29. Tentler, *Catholics and Contraception*, 132.

30. Critchlow, *Intended Consequences*, 13.

31. Ibid.

32. Ibid., 14.

33. Ibid., 112.

34. Ibid.

35. Furedi, *Population and Development*, 73.

36. Ibid., 102.

37. John Paul II, "Letter of His Holiness," par. 3.

38. Ibid., par. 4.

39. Pope Paul VI, *Populorum progressio*, par. 14.

40. Ibid., par. 34.

41. Ibid., par. 36.

42. Ibid., par. 37.

43. Ibid.

44. Ibid., n39.

45. Pope John XXIII, *Mater et magistra*, par. 73.

46. Ibid., par. 189.

47. Ibid.

48. Ibid., par. 194, 199.

49. Pope John Paul II, *Sollicitudo rei socialis*, par. 25.

50. Ibid., par. 25.

51. Ibid.

52. Pope John Paul II, *Familiaris consortio*, par. 30.

53. Ibid., par. 30.

54. Pope Benedict XVI, *Caritas in veritate*, par. 15.

55. Ibid., par. 28.

56. Ibid.

57. Ibid., par. 29.

58. Tentler, *Catholics and Contraception*, 40. For more on John Ryan, see Beckley, *Passion for Justice*, esp. chaps. 3 and 5.

59. This is as quoted by Kennedy, *Birth Control*, 27, from Sanger, *Pivot of Civilization*, 244.

60. Kennedy's biography of Sanger (*Birth Control in America*) is useful, but he depicts her as an overly emotional woman who was unable to retain a consistent outlook throughout her life. Two other books—Angela Franks's *Margaret Sanger's Eugenic Legacy* and Ellen Chesler's *Woman of Valor*—present radically different assessments of Sanger's life. To this day, many valorize Sanger as one of the most influential and courageous women of the twentieth century, but others view her in a strongly negative light.

61. Kennedy, *Birth Control*, xviii.

62. Most feminists have interpreted Sanger's embrace of eugenics as pragmatic. Chesler, for example, writes it off as an "intense desire to have the support of the major secular thinkers of her day." And in another passage, Chesler suggests that Sanger was "caught up in the eugenic zeal of the day" but that her true commitment was to the "overburdened poor"; Chesler, *Woman of Valor,* 216–17. She also dismisses Sanger's eugenics activities as being typical of many progressives of that time. Others, like Franks, have taken a less sympathetic view, arguing that Sanger was ultimately motivated by an ideology of control. Franks writes that "it is essential for women who have admired this pioneer not to be blindly uncritical of her faults and, even more, to realize that she championed an ideology that is much less benign than it first appears, an ideology ultimately destructive of the ideal of female liberation"; Franks, *Margaret Sanger's Eugenic Legacy,* 8.

63. For an example of this type of negative evaluation, see Kennedy, *Birth Control.*

64. Ibid., 176.

65. Ibid., 209.

66. In 1936, the US District Court of Appeals modified the Comstock Act by removing contraceptives from the list of obscene materials that could not be distributed through the mail. Watkins, *On the Pill,* 14.

67. Kennedy, *Birth Control,* 267.

68. Ibid., 141.

69. Ibid., 268.

70. Quoted in ibid., 148.

71. James Cardinal Gibbons, "Pastoral Letter of Cardinal Gibbons on the Celebration of the One Hundredth Anniversary of the Establishment of the Catholic Hierarchy in the United States," 1919, section on marriage, http://cdm.msmary .edu:2011/cdm/ref/collection/Booklets/id/21.

72. Ryan, *Family Limitation,* 3.

73. Ibid., 7.

74. Ibid., 9.

75. Ibid., 13.

76. Ibid., 16.

77. Ibid., 23.

78. Tentler, *Catholics and Contraception,* 41.

79. Ibid.

80. Watkins, *On the Pill,* 14.

81. Ashford, *Resource Flows.*

82. Hartmann, *Reproductive Rights and Wrongs,* 120. Hartmann's book, which was written in 1995, does not mention the Bill & Melinda Gates Foundation, which only became a major player after the mid-1990s.

83. John Paul II, "Letter of His Holiness."

84. Ibid., par. 2.

85. International Conference on Population and Development, "Master Plan."

86. Weigel, writing in *First Things,* stated that "the draft document's view of the human condition and the human prospect was rooted in that concept of the

radically autonomous individual with which Americans have become all too familiar through the sexual revolution, the deconstructionist decay of the American academy, and the philosophical musings of several Supreme Court justices." Weigel, "What Really Happened," 26.

87. The first was held in Bucharest in 1974, and the second in Mexico City in 1984.

88. Rao and Sexton, "Introduction," 4.

89. International Conference on Population and Development, "Master Plan," chap. 3, par. 14.

90. Ibid., chap. 7, par. 13.

91. Ibid., pt. II, chap. 2.

92. Pope John Paul II, "Letter of His Holiness."

# CHAPTER 6

# Conclusion

W HEN I FIRST STARTED researching this book several years ago, the Catholic ethics of contraception seemed like a parochial topic, one that might be of interest only to Catholics. When friends and colleagues would ask what I was working on, I could always count on humorous responses, such as "a book on Catholics and contraception; . . . that ought to take you one page!" What more was there to say about this topic? In the midst of a world that had overwhelmingly accepted the use of contraceptives as a positive, morally licit act, Catholics were the lone holdouts.[1] In other words, debating the morality of contraception seemed somewhat old-fashioned. Even for Catholics, the divisive debates about contraception in the 1960s seemed to have faded, leaving many Catholics to choose privately how they would respond to the Church's ban on artificial contraception. Overwhelmingly, the statistics confirm that many Catholics are using artificial contraception in defiance of the official Church teaching.[2]

By the time I had completed writing most of this book, however, the issue of Catholics and contraception had unexpectedly burst onto the public stage.[3] It reemerged as a contested topic in many public and non-Catholic contexts—most notably in the 2012 US presidential elections. The Catholic teaching about contraception is now at the center of broader political debates about health care, conscience, and freedom of religion. Today it is unlikely that anyone could claim that the morality of contraception is a nonissue; the debate, albeit in a different form than the 1960s, continues to rage. Artificial contraceptives are such a widely accepted part of American culture that the controversies are no longer about their general permissibility, but are rather about whether they ought to be part of the basic provision of health care.

In some ways the recent attention to contraception is really not about contraception at all, but rather about political control.

My choice to pursue this subject matter was not tied to its popularity or lack of popularity. Indeed, I was drawn to it partly because I was puzzled by the lack of scholarly attention to this topic. Since the turbulence of the 1960s, when Americans saw important Supreme Court decisions about contraception followed soon after by Pope Paul VI's *Humanae vitae*, there has been relative silence in the scholarly literature on the morality of contraception. In the intervening years, new issues and developments related to contraceptives convinced me that a close analysis of Catholic moral discourse on contraception would provide an important case to help clarify our understanding of the cultural production of moral arguments. Conversely, I was certain that in order to understand Catholic discourse about contraception, it was necessary to see it as part of broader public practices of moral deliberation. The contexts of HIV/AIDS, rape and emergency contraception, and population require that the discussion about contraception engage with what non-Catholics are saying and doing. Catholic speech about the morality of contraception is always embedded in the overlapping discourses of sex, violence, and justice. These three terms form an inseparable triad insofar as to speak about sexuality is to speak about the violence and harm that it can so easily cause. It is also to speak about just human relationships and about the just social structures necessary to sustain them. My intent throughout this book has been to show how one tradition's responses to a complex issue such as contraception are shaped and molded by cultural realities. I have attempted to suggest some relevant insights about the mechanisms of this culture–religion interaction generally. Indeed, because religious moral discourses engage in practices of public justification, they are deeply cultural expressions.

Contraception is a significant moral issue for numerous reasons, and its significance depends on how one construes this activity. Thus, for some, the morality of artificial contraception is primarily about the regulation of sexual acts and the more particular concern about whether promoting contraception encourages sexual promiscuity. Others construe it mainly as harmful to human life, either directly to an embryo or indirectly through interference with the life-giving process. Yet others worry about the implications of contraception in terms of economic, political, environmental, and gender justice—matters that are tied to the well-being and flourishing of the human community and the planet.

It is noteworthy, yet perhaps not surprising, that people interpret the act of deliberately interfering with human reproduction in such diverse ways. The ethics of human reproduction elicit strong reactions: Exerting control over our procreative capacities imbues humans with a sense of power. Michel Foucault's description of sexuality also applies to contraception. For him, sexuality "appears rather as an especially dense transfer point for relations of power."[4] In other words, it reinforces already unequal power relationships. When people argue for and against artificial contraception, they are essentially offering conflicting accounts of those power arrangements. The decision to regulate births, whether made by individuals or by institutions, is a powerful one. Yet, in this study, we have considered aspects of contraception that are not exclusively about the control of birth. In the contexts of condoms for disease prevention, emergency contraception for rape victims, and economic development, contraception expands to be about more than simply the regulation of births. These contexts suggest a much broader matrix for evaluating the morality of contraception. Foucault also remarks that sexuality is the element of power relations that is "useful for the greatest number of maneuvers and capable of serving as a point of support, as a linchpin, for the most varied strategies."[5] The multifaceted and ubiquitous presence of human sexuality in all power relations complicates any evaluation of contraception. The reemergence of contraception as a central issue in American political discourse in the early twenty-first century testifies to the centrality of sexuality in political arrangements. Recent debates about whether contraception can be mandated as an essential component of health care reform and whether that mandate can be imposed on all citizens regardless of their religious beliefs highlights this dense relationship.

In chapter 1 I identified two goals for this book. First, I wanted the example of one tradition's shaping of moral justifications to offer helpful insights for the study of religious ethics. Second, I hoped that this study would "serve to refresh our view of the relevance of contraception to broader ideas about sex, violence, and justice." Both these goals are ambitious, and I do not presume to have identified radically new insights, but I do believe that my conclusions provide evidence that reinforces and perhaps even expands existing ideas in religious ethics and sexual ethics.

## INSIGHTS FOR RELIGIOUS ETHICS

Religious ethicists can draw two important conclusions about how religious traditions engage in the practice of moral justification from this study. First, religious traditions embody certain sets of practices that facilitate the work of moral deliberation and justification. These are practices captured by the metaphor of negotiation. The term "negotiation" has at least two meanings. One is to aim for an agreement or settlement through conversation, give-and-take, and compromise, as in "our negotiations about where to go for dinner yielded a positive outcome." Another is to accomplish or complete a task, especially one that is difficult or challenging, as in "she negotiated the treacherous mountain path on foot." These two ideas, of conversation aimed at compromise and of the completion of a difficult task, are both central to the practices of moral deliberation. Thus, as we have seen, the Catholic Church's responses to contraception in new contexts require negotiation of both sorts—negotiations that involve theological, cultural, social, and scientific terrains and conversation partners. Through each of the chapters, I have identified the range of "overlapping justifications" the official Catholic discourse utilizes; that is, the grounding of moral arguments through the use of different types of strategies. So, for example, at various times and in various ways, the Catholic tradition appeals to three commandments from the Decalogue. The tradition also alternates between moral and pragmatic appeals. This plurality of approaches stems partly from the fact that contraception, like many other ethical issues, resists categorization. As a result, outlining moral justifications to oppose or support contraceptive practices in the context of a religious tradition will necessarily be a complex activity.

What I think this study suggests more particularly is that this richness of justificatory strategies is both a weakness and a strength of religious traditions. It is a weakness insofar as it can potentially fragment moral discourse and make it difficult for believers and others to understand the reasons for a tradition's moral position. Yet it is also a strength because it acknowledges the interdependence of human practices and institutions. For example, Catholicism's views about contraception are firmly connected to its ideas about the family. In general, the tradition views the family as "an institution of civil society" that is "interdependent with virtually every other" institution.[6] The family's interdependence with every other facet of society means that the morality of procreative decisions and practices is intertwined with a range of moral concerns. Consequently, an issue such as the morality of condom use to prevent disease is both a matter of public health and of sexuality. In the context of HIV/AIDS, the rapid spread of the epidemic is clearly connected to oppressive sexual practices—practices that are reinforced by economic and social inequities. Thus, any attempt to bracket ethical discourse about a particular issue is potentially dangerous because it overlooks these relationships of interdependence. For example, it is dangerous to make the primary concern about condom distribution to prevent HIV/AIDS the promotion of promiscuous behavior, because doing so overlooks serious public health evidence. Conversely, to ignore the role of sexually irresponsible behavior in the spread of the disease would be imprudent. An analogous example of overlapping justifications was evident in the discussion of population in chapter 5. There, the morality of contraception was part of a larger discourse about economic development and justice. Thus, in that context the Church could not limit its appeals simply to sexual morality; it had to characterize contraception as a social justice issue. The difficulties of the debate centered on disagreements about how best to achieve the goals of justice and equality.

The second conclusion relevant to religious ethics pertains to the question of change and development in religious traditions. This is an issue of great interest to those who study moral traditions. It has become commonplace to note that traditions, as vibrant, living entities, must change in order to survive. But how do we evaluate these changes? Are certain changes more authentic than others? For example, are changes that result from pressures internal to a tradition somehow more real and true than changes that result from external ones? At what point is a religious tradition simply giving in and conforming to the surrounding culture? We might also ponder whether there is a limit to how much change a tradition can withstand. This study offers some insight on these matters. In the context of Catholicism, change is an especially vexed issue tied to questions of objectivity and authority. The case of condoms discussed in chapter 3 provides one example of the variety of pressures on a tradition to change. We saw that the pressures emerge *both* from within and outside the tradition. This combined force appears to be succeeding: at this point, many signs point toward a reversal of the teaching on this particular issue. As noted in earlier chapters, Pope Francis appears to be sympathetic to allowing the use of condoms as part of disease prevention efforts. If he does alter the teaching, we might expect him to appeal to external scientific evidence. Yet he will also have a wide range of possible justifications at his disposal, as well as the rich tradition of casuistical tools (e.g., double effect, toleration, and proportionality) to which many Catholic theologians have already appealed. One can presume that this will enable the Church to make an adjustment without undermining the integrity of the tradition.

The concept of tradition is deployed differently in the case of emergency contraception and rape. The US Catholic bishops' directive about allowing emergency contraception for rape victims relies on a long-standing view that rape is unjust aggression and thus the rapist's sperm is an unjust aggressor. Whereas in the case of the morality of condoms, tradition offers numerous theoretical resources for expansion and amendment; in this case it offers a precise and direct line of teaching between the bishops' directive and Sanchez's teaching about the expulsion of semen. Yet our discussion of the rich history of exceptional cases in chapter 4 raised questions about whether this way of viewing traditions only focuses on aspects of tradition that are convenient for maintaining authority. In other words, decisions about which cases count and about who has the authority to decide matter greatly. The pressure for change on this issue comes primarily from Catholics who would argue that this very narrow set of circumstances—women who have been raped and are able to get to an emergency room within 72 hours—is no different from cases of women who seek out emergency contraception for other reasons. In other words, they question whether rape victims should constitute a separate category. This is a matter that is further complicated by the underlying issue of how one defines what counts as sex.

The Catholic responses to contraception in the context of economic development and globalization in chapter 5 point to another aspect of the deployment of tradition. The Church's teachings about population control in these contexts have always been connected to its tradition of thought about social justice. As we saw, the papal encyclicals by John XXIII, Paul VI, John Paul II, and Benedict XVI all emphasize the links between families, development, and moral order. Thus, they all argue that development of peoples must always be "integral." An undue focus on one aspect of the common good at the expense of others is a distortion of the demands of justice. Unlike the other two cases, contraception, when viewed in the context of the discourse of population control, appeals to a very different aspect of the Catholic tradition—an aspect focused on social, scientific, and economic policies.

## SEX, VIOLENCE, AND JUSTICE

The second goal I identified in chapter 1 concerns how this study might refresh our ideas about sex, violence, and gender. On the issue of sex, it is noteworthy that a central concern of the early "birth control" movement in nineteenth-century America was a perception that sexual immorality was on the rise. As Peter Engelman notes about the period after the Civil War, "war-torn America had been fertile ground for sexual commerce, which continued to thrive after the war."[7] Many have perceived this environment as one of vice and degradation that was especially harmful to women. As a response, the emerging women's temperance and suffrage movements joined forces with Protestant moral reformers to battle what they saw as a "moral crisis in the nation's cities." Engelman describes their motivation as follows: "By restricting sexual expression to the home, purity crusaders hoped to reassert the reproductive function of sexuality and the spiritual nature of the marriage bond."[8] Although their main targets were the regulation of prostitution and obscenity, they also focused on contraception because they believed that "it further drove the divide between sex for reproduction and sex for pleasure."[9] In this one historical example, we can see how worries about sexual excess and immorality often drive the discourses of contraception.

This connection between sexual immorality and contraception persists in the contemporary Catholic discourse about contraception. The case of condoms and HIV/AIDS is the most obvious example of this connection; yet that case also complicates an easy correlation between sexual immorality and contraception. From a public health perspective, the primary concern with HIV/AIDS prevention ought to be its effectiveness, and we saw that many of the official Catholic statements affirm that point. Yet, much of the Catholic discourse about condoms is shaped by a perception that condoms encourage sexual promiscuity. This anxiety can be characterized as a type of slippery-slope thinking whereby acceptance of condoms by married couples infected with HIV is seen as condoning sexual acts that are not procreative. The point is that sexual practices are always implicated in wider social structures.

Divorcing them from these structures leads to distorted moral analysis, a point that all three cases in this study reinforce. Moreover, this distortion further obscures implicit ideas about justice. This matters, because discourses of sexual morality, or chastity in Catholic terms, that fail to account for protection from harm and the elimination of injustice are bound to be incomplete and potentially dangerous.

## NEGOTIATING CONTESTED TERRAIN

Another way to organize the insights that this case study offers is in terms of what we might learn about how we understand, conceptualize, and negotiate a range of important social and scholarly "terrains" such as history, gender, the body and sexual practices, and politics and authority. One aspect of traditions that many find appealing is that they seem to present a unified front and thus are able to provide consistent and objective answers to moral dilemmas. In the context of a pro or con stance on contraception, the official Catholic position has certainly been consistent. Nevertheless, some have argued that the Church's approval of natural family planning in the 1950s was a sign of inconsistency; whereas others saw it as a sign of development and a deepening of the tradition. Regardless of the point about consistency, the historical trajectory of the Catholic discourse about contraception is burdened by its implication in other discourses about the meaning of marriage, the acceptability of magic and potions, the distinction between natural and unnatural, and the ethics of mutilation. John Noonan's insights about the different types of justifications that have been used to ground the Catholic prohibition against contraception provided us with a helpful guide to this history. They enabled us to connect the discourses about contraception firmly to the Catholic practice of categorizing sins in relation to the Ten Commandments.

This study has also raised questions about how we conceptualize and use the category of gender. As Joan Scott notes, gender helps feminist scholars to better understand "the social organization of the relationship between the sexes."[10] How is contraception gendered? How do contraceptive acts organize and influence these social relations? Can a gender analysis help us negotiate questions about the official Catholic understanding of the use of condoms for disease prevention, its views about rape and contraception, or its population control policies? The answers to these questions are implicit throughout this study. Contraception is a gendered practice for many obvious reasons. The process of procreation implicates women's bodies and lives more directly than those of men; thus, women's ability to regulate conception is especially important. Men also have much to gain or lose from contraception insofar as it allows them to have sex with fewer worries about its consequences. That birth control can liberate women and make them less dependent on men has been a long-standing reason for the feminist embrace of increased access to contraception. In addition to the inherently gendered nature of the issue, the Catholic discourse on sex is clearly gendered. We see this in everything from the continued hold that the doctrine of gender complementarity has on Church teaching to the view still held by many Catholic moralists that a truly marital sex act must involve male ejaculation in the woman's vagina. The view of the woman's body as a receptacle reinforces female objectification and highlights the importance of gendered roles in the construction of Catholic sexual ethics.

This relates to another central concern of this study: the construction of the body and of sexual practices. In order to fully understand this construction, we need to reflect on the relationship between biological reality and socially embedded reality. How is the Catholic vision of contraceptive practices shaped by specific attitudes about the meaning and purposes of the human body? The history of Catholic sexual ethics is characterized by a move from seeing procreation as the primary (and in some cases only) purpose of sex, to acknowledging that other purposes might be equally important. The idea of equal and inseparable purposes that has emerged in modern Catholic moral theology ensures that the body is always seen first and foremost in its biological reality.

The centrality of the body as biological reality is also evident in another context. Pope John Paul II reflects on the relationship between marriage and celibacy—a relationship that might appear at first to be quite distant from the concerns surrounding the morality of contraception. He claims that it is only through a strong respect for celibacy that strong marriage can exist. For him, the example of celibate humans teaches all people the discipline of bodily control, and this discipline is necessary because it is a central component even in marriage. That sexual practices must be disciplined is an underlying theme of Catholic discourses about contraception which often connect contraception to a lack of self-discipline. Thus, though celibacy embodies self-discipline in a pure and exemplary way, the Church also teaches that marital sexuality ought to strive to achieve a similar goal. These ideas about the biological reality of sex and gender, as well as the emphasis on self-discipline, are reinforced by the theological idea that marriage is a sacrament. To say that marriage is a sacrament is to say that it enacts something real and embodied; it is not a symbol. Hence, just as the Eucharist is for Catholics the real body and blood of Christ, marriage is the real marriage of Christ and Church. The consummation of marriage has a sacral character; the physical and the spiritual are intermingled. Thus, ideas about the body in Catholic teaching are grounded in ideas about its biological reality. Nevertheless, these ideas are at their core profoundly theological.

On a more practical level, negotiating contraception brings us face-to-face with concerns about the moral and epistemic grounding of authority. Margaret Walker describes feminist ethics as aspiring "toward transparency" in moral life—an ideal that "is at once a moral and epistemic one."[11] As I noted in chapter 1, she believes that feminist ethics contributes to our understanding of ethics by challenging "epistemic and moral authority that is politically engineered and self-reinforcing." This description of authority characterizes Catholic discourses about contraception. Our study of the various contexts in which that discourse is deployed provides critics with material for understanding this engineering. The question of who has the ultimate authority to decide about these issues is at the heart of any inquiry of religious ethics. If we view sexuality in Foucault's terms as a transfer point for relations of power, we can see how the control of the procreative outcomes of sexuality extends that transference. Women's desires to control their reproductive capacities are clearly tied to broader questions of agency and authority.

The final contested terrain that this study sheds light on is the political. The question of who has authority (legal, legislative, economic) over procreation, as well as the related question of what it means to have authority over procreation, has serious political implications as can be seen in US debates about health care reform and the Catholic responses to the "contraceptive mandate" in 2012–13. The controversy sparked by the federal government's announcement in 2012 that it would require contraceptive coverage without copays or deductibles as part of all employer-provided health insurance highlighted these political implications. Some Catholics perceived this move as an attempt to force Catholic employers to act in ways that violated their moral values. In the following final section I attend to the debates that the "contraceptive mandate" elicited to see how they might further illuminate the political implications of this study.

## THE "CONTRACEPTIVE MANDATE"

It is difficult to identify an exact beginning to the public debate about the "contraceptive mandate." For much of the period 2009–11, Americans were eagerly following the legislative attempts to fashion an adequate health care plan that would extend coverage to citizens who were not covered by any health insurance. The process was not an easy one, as there was a wide cultural divide between those who advocated for as much coverage as possible for the most underprivileged and those who were concerned about too much government intervention in health care. The US Catholic bishops, inspired by a long-standing commitment to social justice, were advocating for extending coverage to the underprivileged as long as the coverage did not violate Catholic principles.[12] Thus, in the initial phases of the debate, the matter of reproductive services was not a significant part of the public discourse on health care reform.

Most Americans only began to make the connection between contraception and health care reform when the Institute of Medicine's (IOM) July 2011 recommendations deemed that all health insurance plans ought to be required to cover contraception, sterilization, and reproductive education services at no cost to the patient. The IOM was commissioned by the Department of Health and Human Services "to conduct a review of effective preventive services to ensure women's health and well-being."[13] This review was part of the broader discussions about the overhaul of the nation's health care system that was envisioned by the Patient Protection and Affordable Care Act (ACA) passed by the US Congress in 2010. The ACA emphasizes the importance of making preventive services and screenings available to millions of Americans.

The IOM report identified a set of recommendations based on what the panel saw as gaps in the provision of preventive services for women. In looking at the particular health needs of American women, the IOM identified eight general areas—most of which received little scrutiny from the public. The report's insistence that contraception was a preventive health service that ought to be provided as part of the ACA to all women free of charge generated much controversy and propelled the issue of contraception into the public light. The report characterized "unintended pregnancy" as a "health condition," and thus deemed that "family planning services" could be considered as medically "preventive services" and would thus be required.[14]

Daniel Cardinal DiNardo, chairman of the Committee on Pro-Life Activities of the US Conference of Catholic Bishops, responded on behalf of the Church to the IOM recommendation in 2011. His response provides a summary of the range of justifications we have covered in this study. DiNardo identifies three items on the IOM's list of preventive health services as ones that the Catholic Church could not accept: surgical sterilization, all birth control approved by the Food and Drug Administration (including emergency contraception), and education and counseling that would promote birth control. He appeals to several types of arguments that focus mostly on concerns about justice and harm to the fetus. Interestingly, he does not mention the harm to marriage, or the link between increased access to contraception and sexual promiscuity, concerns that are central to most official Catholic discourse about contraception. Rather, DiNardo is more concerned about the IOM report's framing of pregnancy as something to be prevented. He writes: "Pregnancy is not a disease, and fertility is not a pathological condition to be suppressed by any means technically possible." In the background, of course, is his concern about abortion, especially about how this mandate might pave the way for a similar mandate about surgical abortions. As we have seen at various points in this study, this connection between abortion and contraception is common in Catholic discourse. Finally, DiNardo also expresses concern about several issues that could loosely be grouped together as concerns about justice. One is a worry that directing attention and funding to contraception diverts important resources from other more pressing matters such as immigration and poverty. This type of appeal is an example of the centrality of the common good in Catholic social thought. Bishop DiNardo also expresses concern about justice in a very different way. He is worried that requiring all citizens to pay for contraceptive services will require many to violate deeply held values and beliefs. As he states: "The considerable cost of these practices will be paid by all who participate in health coverage."[15]

This report was only the beginning of what came to be ongoing public relations, political, and legal battles between official representatives of the Catholic Church and the administration of President Obama. In the wake of the IOM report, Obama issued a directive that required all health insurance plans to cover contraceptive services for women. He did, however, allow for a narrow exemption for religious institutions that were morally opposed to contraception. This exemption did not include institutions such as hospitals, universities, and nonprofits that were administered by religious denominations but served and employed non-Catholics. The US Conference of Catholic Bishops responded by claiming that such a narrow definition of religious institutions was a violation of religious freedom. Supporters of Obama, by contrast, saw this as a reasonable accommodation. Indeed, some were worried that even the limited accommodation might be an unfair imposition of religious teaching on nonreligious employees of these institutions. Some American Catholics and many others responded with great alarm and passion when in February 2012, the Obama administration announced that it was going to require Catholic institutions (with the exception of churches) to comply with this mandate. Though some responses were based on concerns about the morality of contraception, many were about the government's reach in requiring institutions to act in ways that violated their stated moral doctrines. This led many to appeal to freedom of conscience and to argue that it violated the US constitution to require religious institutions to participate in an activity that they deemed immoral. They claimed that even if Catholic institutions were not directly providing contraception or encouraging employees to use it, they were still morally implicated in an immoral act. In terms of Catholic principles, they were "cooperating with evil."[16]

The principle of cooperation with evil is a long-standing Catholic principle that traditionally has been used to determine the extent of a person's culpability in moral wrongdoing. Cathleen Kaveny's recent detailed analysis of this principle illustrates both its importance and the confusion that often surrounds its proper interpretation. She explains that cooperation with evil emerged as an important concept in the context of the pre–Vatican II manuals of moral theology that were composed to help confessors negotiate individual human sins. In that context, cooperation with evil was viewed as an individual act rather than as a category that could describe an institution. For example, manualists discuss cases such as "whether a cab driver can deliver a customer to a house of prostitution, whether a head-of-household can work at a munitions plant for making weapons of mass destruction, and whether a physician or a counselor can refer a patient for an abortion."[17]

Moralists further distinguish cooperation with evil along the lines of formal and material·cooperation. The distinction between formal and material rests largely on the agent's intention vis-à-vis the wrongdoing, since in both cases the effects of an action are foreseen. Formal cooperation, which involves cases when "the cooperator agrees either with the evil moral object of the act (*finis operis*) or with the evil intention (*finis operantis*) of the principal agent," is always forbidden.[18] Material cooperation, which can be acceptable in certain cases, encompasses situations where the agent might foresee the evil of the act but does not intend it. In other words, he or she contributes to, or in some way facilitates, the action, but "the cooperator neither intends the object of the act nor agrees with the intention of the principal agent."[19] Critics of the Catholic Bishops claimed the Obama mandate, especially in its revised forms, would in no way implicate Catholics in formal cooperation. David Gibson writes that "the contraception battle, like most ethical dilemmas, is more focused on 'material' cooperation. This means you neither approve of an action nor want it to occur, so you take steps to separate yourself as much as possible from the action."[20] The tradition allows for great latitude in the evaluation of cases of material cooperation.

Kaveny clarifies the conversation about cooperation with evil by making two important points. Her first point is that the term "intrinsic evil" is often carelessly tossed about in contemporary Catholic debates without any real understanding of what the tradition of Catholic moral theology really intended by the term. She writes: "It is not a rhetorical flourish; instead, it is a highly technical term of Catholic moral theology with roots in scripture as well as in the action theory of St. Thomas Aquinas."[21] The misuse and overuse of the term have led to her second point; that labeling everything remotely related to evil as "intrinsic evil" diminishes the force of the category and fails to offer any real guidance about how to respond to it. Moreover, it makes drawing any meaningful lines very difficult. She writes: "If every foreseen and foreseeable consequence of the act of voting rises to the level of a cooperation with evil problem, then virtually every other act an agent performs entails a similar cooperation with evil problem."[22] Kaveny's concern is that it would be possible to expand the principle of cooperation to such a degree that it would eclipse an important distinction between "the background conditions of original sin and human sociality" and cooperation with evil.[23] The issue of whether Catholic employers are being forced to cooperate with evil when their employees receive federally mandated contraceptive coverage is thus more complex than the US Catholic bishops suggest. Gibson's point reminds us about the importance of the formal/material discussion and Kaveny warns us about the serious implications that result from the misuse of these categories.

In February 2013, the Obama administration issued a revised position that expanded the exemption to include hospitals, universities, and nonprofit charities that are administered by religious institutions. This seeming compromise was not embraced by all because many hoped that the administration would extend the exemption to include all religious believers, even secular business owners who would be required to provide contraceptive coverage to all their employees.[24] The intricacies of this debate are complex, mainly because the issue of contraception itself was often either overlooked or conflated with religious liberty, freedom of conscience, and cooperation with evil issues. Thus while the recent "contraceptive mandate" debates brought the issue of contraception to the forefront, they often ignored the moral arguments about whether or not artificial contraception is morally licit.

Nevertheless, these public policy debates remind us both that the moral issues surrounding contraception are far from settled and that the issue of contraception is a moving target. Indeed, we can see it as embodying societal anxieties about the various "terrains" discussed earlier in this chapter. While this study does not settle the many moral complexities surrounding contraception, it does highlight an important point; that like many moral issues, contraception must be understood as nested within a group of issues that are shaped by cultural forces. Thus, decisions about whether or not to use contraception are always necessarily connected to beliefs about appropriate sexual practices, to our desire to protect ourselves from bodily harm, and to our need to live in a just society. Negotiating the moral issue of contraception requires attention to these complex interconnections.

# NOTES

1. Most Protestant denominations had accepted the use of artificial contraceptives by the 1970s. Tom Davis's interesting study of religious involvement in Planned Parenthood in the United States describes the extent of that acceptance. See Davis, *Sacred Work*.

2. There has been some controversy about the surveys and polls that claim that up to 98 percent of sexually active Catholic women have used contraceptive means not approved by the Church. However, several studies indicate that even if not 98 percent, the numbers are fairly high.

3. Jana Bennett expresses this sentiment when she writes that "there is no way—no WAY—I would have thought that the Church's teaching against contraception would see anything like the national stage that it received in January and February." Bennett, "2012: In the US, the Year of Catholic Moral Theology?"

4. Foucault, *History of Sexuality*, 103.

5. Ibid.

6. Cahill, *Family*, 7.

7. Engelman, *History of the Birth Control Movement*, 13.

8. Ibid., 14.

9. Ibid.

10. Scott, "Gender," 1053.

11. Walker, *Moral Understandings*, 79.

12. See, e.g., the letter from the US Catholic bishops to the US House of Representatives sent on January 26, 2010. They write: "The Catholic bishops have long supported adequate and affordable health care for all, because health care is a basic human right. As pastors and teachers, we believe genuine health care reform must protect human life and dignity, not threaten them, especially for the most voiceless and vulnerable. We believe health care legislation must respect the consciences of providers, taxpayers, and others, not violate them. We believe universal coverage should be truly universal and should not be denied to those in need because of their condition, age, where they come from, or when they arrive here. Providing affordable and accessible health care that clearly reflects these fundamental principles is a public good, moral imperative, and urgent national priority." This passage illustrates that while they are concerned about the content of the health care legislation, they support the view that health care is a basic right. The letter is available at www.usccb.org/issues-and-action/human-life-and-dignity/health-care/upload/health-care-letter-to-congress-2010–01–26.pdf.

13. Institute of Medicine, "Clinical Preventive Services," 1.

14. Ibid., 104.

15. US Conference of Catholic Bishops, July 19, 2011.

16. See David Cloutier's article in the days following the Obama administration's announcement. He identifies the main issues that concerned many Catholics and also raises some interesting questions about the applicability of "cooperation with evil" to this context. Cloutier, "Mandate."

17. Kaveny, *Law's Virtues*, 246–47.

18. Catholic Health Care Association, "Principles Governing Cooperation," 25.

19. Ibid., 25–26. For more on the distinctions between various types of cooperation, see Kaveny, "Appropriation of Evil"; Kaveny and Keenan, "Ethical Issues";
and Sulmasy, "Catholic Participation in Needle- and Syringe-Exchange Programs."

20. Gibson, "Contraception Objections Fail."

21. Kaveny, *Law's Virtues*, 220.

22. Ibid., 252. In this discussion, Kaveny is writing about the use of the terms
"intrinsic evil" and "cooperation with evil" in the context of whether Catholics can
morally vote for prochoice political candidates.

23. Ibid.

24. For an articulation of the continued opposition to the Obama administration position, see US Conference of Catholic Bishops, "USCCB Says Administration Mandate Violates First Amendment."

# BIBLIOGRAPHY

Allen, John J., Jr., and Pamela Schaeffer. "Reports of Abuse: AIDS Exacerbates Sexual Exploitation of Nuns, Reports Allege." *National Catholic Reporter*, March 16, 2001. www.natcath.com?NCR_On line/archives/031601/031601a.htm.

Aquinas, Thomas. *On the Sentences.*

———. *Summa Contra Gentiles.*

———. *Summa Theologiae.* Excerpted in *Saint Thomas Aquinas on Law, Morality, and Politics*, edited by William P. Baumgarth and Richard J. Regan, SJ. Indianapolis: Hackett, 1988.

Ashford, Lori. *Resource Flows for International Population Assistance and UNFPA.* Washington, DC: Center for Global Development, 2010. www.cgdev.org/doc/Resources-at-UNFPA.pdf.

Augustine, Saint. *City of God*, translated by Henry Bettenson. London: Penguin Books, 2003.

———. *Confessions*, translated by Henry Chadwick. Oxford: Oxford University Press, 1981.

———. *Treatise on Marriage and Other Subjects* (*The Fathers of the Early Church*), edited by Charles T. Wilcox, MM, and Roy J. Deferarri. Washington, DC: Catholic University of America Press, 1955.

Austriaco, OP, and Nicanor Pier Giorgio. "Is Plan B an Abortifacient? A Critical Look at the Scientific Evidence." *National Catholic Bioethics Quarterly* 7, no. 4 (2007): 703–7.

Barragán, Javier Cardinal Lozano. "Message on the Occasion of World AIDS Day." Pontifical Council for Health Pastoral Care, December 1, 2005. www.vatican.va/roman_curia/pontifical_councils/hlthwork/documents/rc_pc_hlthwor.

Baumgarth, William P., and Richard J. Regan, SJ, eds. *Saint Thomas Aquinas on Law, Morality, and Politics.* Indianapolis: Hackett, 1988.

Bayer, Edward, STD. *Rape within Marriage: A Moral Analysis Delayed.* New York: University Press of America, 1985.

Beckley, Harlan. *Passion for Justice: Retrieving the Legacies of Walter Rauschenbusch, John A. Ryan, and Reinhold Niebuhr.* Louisville: Westminster / John Knox Press, 1992.

Benedict XVI, Pope. *Caritas in veritate,* 2009.

———. "Interview of the Holy Father Benedict XVI in Preparation for the Apostolic Journey to Bavaria." August 2006. Available at www.vatican.va.

———. *Light of the World: The Pope, the Church, and the Signs of the Times—A Conversation with Peter Seewald.* San Francisco: Ignatius Press, 2010.

Bennett, Jana. "2012: In the US, the Year of Catholic Moral Theology?" December 25, 2012. http://catholicmoraltheology.com/2012-in-the-us-the-year-of-catholic-moral-theology.

Bouchard, Charles E., and James R. Pollock. "Condoms and the Common Good." *Second Opinion* 12 (1989): 98–106.

Brunton, Jennifer, CNM, MSN, and Margaret W. Beal, CNM. "Current Issues in Emergency Contraception: An Overview for Providers." *Journal of Midwifery and Women's Health* 51, no. 6 (November–December 2006).

Bucar, Elizabeth M. *Creative Conformity: The Feminist Politics of US Catholic and Iranian Shi'i Women.* Washington, DC: Georgetown University Press, 2011.

Cahill, Lisa Sowle. "AIDS, Justice, and the Common Good." In *Catholic Ethicists on HIV/AIDS Prevention,* edited by James F. Keenan, SJ. London: Continuum, 2000.

———. *Family: A Christian Social Perspective.* Minneapolis: Fortress Press, 2000.

———. *Sex, Gender, and Christian Ethics.* Cambridge: Cambridge University Press, 1996.

———. *Theological Bioethics: Participation, Justice and Change.* Washington, DC: Georgetown University Press, 2005.

Cahill, Lisa Sowle, Jon Fuller, James Keenan, Kevin Kelly, Enda McDonagh, and Robert Vitillo, eds. *Catholic Ethicists on HIV/AIDS Prevention.* New York: Continuum, 2000.

Callahan, Daniel, ed. *The Catholic Case for Contraception.* New York: Macmillan, 1969.

Calvin, John. *Institutes of the Christian Religion,* edited by John T. McNeill. Philadelphia: Westminster Press, 1960.

Cardegna, Felix F., SJ. "Contraception, the Pill, and Responsible Parenthood." *Theological Studies* 25, no. 4 (December 1964).

Cates, Diana Fritz. *Aquinas on the Emotions: A Religious-Ethical Inquiry.* Washington, DC: Georgetown University Press, 2009.

Catholic Health Care Association. "The Principles Governing Cooperation and Catholic Health Care: An Overview." www.chausa.org/docs/default-source/general-files/a7ca2015424c4be8b14e998250 58c8931-pdf.pdf?sfvrsn=0.

CELAM Office of Justice and Solidarity. "Pastoral Strategy on HIV and AIDS." Consejo Episcopal Latinoamericano, December 2005. www.caritas.org/includes/pdf/ReportToXVIIIAssembly.pdf.

Chesler, Ellen. *Woman of Valor: Margaret Sanger and the Birth Control Movement in America.* New York: Simon & Schuster, 2007.

*Christian Century.* "Morning-After Pill OK." June 18–25, 1986.

Cloutier, David. "The Mandate: Three Lessons So Far." February 12, 2012. http://catholicmoraltheology.com/the-mandate-three-lessons-so-far/.

Code of Canon Law. www.vatican.va/archive/eng1104/_index.htm.

Coeytaux, Francine, and Barbara Pillsbury. "Bringing Emergency Contraception to American Women: The History and Remaining Challenges." *Women's Health Issues* 11, no. 2 (March–April 2001).

Cohen-Kohler, J. C. "The Morally Uncomfortable Global Drug Gap." *Clinical Pharmacology and Therapeutics* 82, no. 5 (November 2007): 610–14. www.ncbi.nlm.nih.gov/pubmed/17898710.

Congregation for the Doctrine of Faith. *Dignitas personae (On Certain Bioethical Questions).* Vatican City: Congregation for the Doctrine of Faith, 2008. www.vatican.va/roman_curia/congregations/cfaith/documents/rc_con_cfaith_doc_20081208_dignitas-personae_en.html.

Connery, John, SJ. *Abortion: The Development of the Roman Catholic Perspective.* Chicago: Loyola University Press, 1977.

———. "Notes on Moral Theology." *Theological Studies* 20, no. 4 (December 1959): 628.

Critchlow, Donald T. *Intended Consequences: Birth Control, Abortion, and the Federal Government in Modern America.* Oxford: Oxford University Press, 1999.

Cross, F. L., ed. *The Oxford Dictionary of the Christian Church.* London: Oxford University Press, 1958.

Croxatto, Horatio, and Soledad Diaz Fernandez. "Emergency Contraception: A Human Rights Issue." *Best Practice and Research Clinical Obstetrics and Gynaecology* 20, no. 3 (2005).

Curran, Charles. *Catholic Moral Theology in the United States: A History.* Washington, DC: Georgetown University Press, 2008.

———. *The Catholic Moral Tradition Today: A Synthesis.* Washington, DC: Georgetown University Press, 1999.

———. *Catholic Social Teaching 1891–Present: A Historical, Theological, and Ethical Analysis.* Washington, DC: Georgetown University Press, 2002.

———. *Dialogue about Catholic Sexual Teaching*, edited by Charles E. Curran and Richard A. McCormick. New York: Paulist Press, 1993.

Davis, Tom. *Sacred Work: Planned Parenthood and Its Clergy Alliances.* New Brunswick, NJ: Rutgers University Press, 2005.

Decter, Midge. "The Nine Lives of Population Control." In *The 9 Lives of Population Control*, edited by Michael Cromartie. Grand Rapids: William B. Eerdmans, 1995.

Dulles, Avery. "The Church." In *The Documents of Vatican II*, edited by Walter M. Abbott, SJ. New York: America Press, 1966.

Ehrlich, Paul R. *The Population Bomb.* New York: Ballantine Books, 1968.

Engelman, Peter C. *A History of the Birth Control Movement in America.* Santa Barbara, CA: Praeger, 2011.

Ewig, Christina. "Hijacking Global Feminism: Feminists, the Catholic Church, and the Family Planning Debacle in Peru." *Feminist Studies* 32, no. 3 (Fall 2006): 633–59.

Farley, Margaret A. *Just Love: A Framework for Christian Sexual Ethics.* New York: Continuum, 2006.

———. "Partnership in Hope: Gender, Faith, and Responses to HIV/AIDS in Africa." *Journal of Feminist Studies in Religion* 20, no. 1 (Spring 2004): 133–48.

Farmer, Paul, and David Walton. "Condoms, Coups and the Ideology of Prevention: Facing Failure in Rural Haiti." In *Catholic Ethicists on HIV/AIDS Prevention*, edited by James F. Keenan, SJ. New York: Continuum, 2000.

Farraher, Joseph F., SJ. "Notes on Moral Theology." *Theological Studies* 24, no. 1 (March 1963).

Farrow, Alexandra, M. G. R. Hull, K. Northstone, H. Taylor, W. C. L. Ford, and J. Golding. "Prolonged Use of Oral Contraception before a Planned Pregnancy Is Associated with a Decreased Risk of Delayed Conception." *Human Reproduction* 17, no. 10 (2002): 2754–61.

Faúndes, Anibal, Luis Tavara, Vivian Brache, and Frank Alvarez. "Emergency Contraception under Attack in Latin America; Response of the Medical Establishment and Civil Society." *Reproductive Health Matters* 15, no. 29 (2007).

Foucault, Michel. *The History of Sexuality: An Introduction*, vol. 1. Translated by Robert Hurley. New York: Vintage Books, 1990.

Franks, Angela. *Margaret Sanger's Eugenic Legacy: The Control of Female Fertility*. Jefferson, NC: McFarland, 2005.

Fuchs, Joseph, SJ. *Moral Demands and Personal Obligations*. Washington, DC: Georgetown University Press, 1993.

Fuller, Jon D., SJ, and James F. Keenan, SJ. "Introduction: At the End of the First Generation of HIV Prevention." In *Catholic Ethicists on HIV/AIDS Prevention*, edited by James F. Keenan, SJ. London: Continuum, 2000.

Furedi, Frank. *Population and Development: A Critical Introduction*. Cambridge: Polity Press, 1997.

Gallagher, John. "Magisterial Teaching from 1918 to the Present." In *Dialogue about Catholic Sexual Teaching*, edited by Charles E. Curran and Richard A. McCormick. New York: Paulist Press, 1993.

———. *Time Past, Time Future: An Historical Study of Catholic Moral Theology*. New York: Paulist Press, 1990.

Gemzell-Danielsson, Kristina, Cecilia Berger, and P. G. L. Lalitkumar. "Emergency Contraception: Mechanisms of Action." *Contraception* 87 (2013): 305.

Genilo, Eric Marcelo O., SJ. *John Cuthbert Ford, SJ: Moral Theologian at the End of the Manualist Era*. Washington, DC: Georgetown University Press, 2007.

Gibson, David. "Contraception Objections Fail Catholic's Moral Reasoning." *USA Today*, February 14, 2012.

Glasier, Anna. "Emergency Contraception: Clinical Outcomes." *Contraception* 87 (2013): 310.

Goldberg, Michelle. *The Means of Reproduction: Sex, Power, and the Future of the World*. New York: Penguin, 2009.

Gomez, Jim, and Tim Sullivan. "'7 Billionth' Babies Feted, as Is OC's Baby Jay." *Orange County Register*, October 31, 2011. www.ocregister.com/news/billion-324644-population-born.html.

Grabowski, John. *Sex and Virtue: An Introduction to Sexual Ethics*. Washington, DC: Catholic University of America Press, 2003.

Grant, Robert. "Review of Contraception by John T. Noonan." *Journal of Religion* 46, no. 2 (April 1966): 304–30.

Gress, Carrie. "AIDS in Africa: Abstinence Works—Interview with Expert Matthew Hanley." *Zenit*, February 27, 2008. www.zenit.org/article-21909?!=english.

Grisez, Germain. *Contraception and the Natural Law.* Milwaukee: Bruce, 1964.

———. "Moral Questions on Condoms and Disease Prevention." *National Catholic Bioethics Quarterly* 8, no. 3 (Autumn 2008): 471–76.

———. *The Way of the Lord Jesus: Moral Principles.* Quincy, IL: Franciscan Press, 1997.

Grisez, Germain, Joseph Boyle, John Finnis, and William E. May. "NFP: Not Contralife." In *The Teaching of "Humane Vitae": A Defense.* San Francisco: Ignatius Press, 1988.

Gudorf, Christine. "Catholicism, Twentieth and Twenty-First-Century." In *Sex from Plato to Paglia: A Philosophical Encyclopedia*, edited by Alan Soble. Westport, CT: Greenwood Press, 2006.

———. "Encountering the Other: The Modern Papacy on Women." *Social Compass* 36, no. 3 (1989): 295–310.

Guevin, Benedict, OSB, and Martin Rhonheimer. "On the Use of Condoms to Prevent Acquired Immune Deficiency Syndrome." *National Catholic Bioethics Quarterly* 5, no. 1 (Spring 2005): 37–48.

Gula, Richard, SS. *Reason Informed by Faith: Foundations of Catholic Morality.* New York: Paulist Press, 1989.

Hamel, Ronald, and Michael Panicola. "Emergency Contraception and Sexual Assault: Assessing the Moral Approaches in Catholic Teaching." *Health Progress* 83, no. 5 (September–October 2002): 12–19.

Hardon, John A. *Modern Catholic Dictionary.* Garden City, NY: Doubleday, 1980.

Häring, Bernard. "Commandments, Ten." In *The New Catholic Encyclopedia*, vol. 4, 5–8. New York: McGraw Hill, 1967.

Hartmann, Betsy. *Reproductive Rights and Wrongs: The Global Politics of Population Control*, rev. ed. Boston: South End Press, 1995.

Hoose, Bernard. *Proportionalism: The American Debate and Its European Roots.* Washington, DC: Georgetown University Press, 1987.

Institute of Medicine. "Clinical Preventive Services for Women: Closing the Gaps." July 19, 2011. http://iom.edu/Reports/2011/Clinical-Preventive-Services-for-Women-Closing-the-Gaps.aspx.

Interdicasterial Commission for the *Catechism of the Catholic Church.* *Catechism of the Catholic Church.* Mahwah, NJ: Paulist Press (Libreria Editrice Vaticana), 1994.

International Conference on Population and Development. "Master Plan: Programme of Action." 1994. www.unfpa.org/public/cache/offonce/home/sitemap/icpd/International-Conference-on-Popula tion-and-Development/ICPD-Programme;jsessionid = E17A04B 72B76BB3DDA3D7A2653F6DD67.jahia01#ch3b.

Jerome, Saint. *Select Letters of St. Jerome*, with an English translation by F. A. Wright. Cambridge, MA: Harvard University Press, 1954.

John Paul II, Pope. "Address to HE Ms. Monique Patricia Antoinette Frank, Ambassador of the Kingdom of the Netherlands to the Holy See." January 22, 2005. www.vatican.va/holy_father/john_paul_ii/speeches/2005/january/documents/hf_jp-ii_spe_20050122_ambas sador-netherlands_en.html.

———. *Evangelium vitae* (*The Gospel of Life*). New York: Random House, 1995.

———. *Familiaris consortio.* 1981.

———. "Letter of His Holiness John Paul II to the Secretary-General of the International Conference on Population and Development." March 18, 1994. www.vatican.va/holy_father/john_paul_ii/letters/1994/documents/hf_jp-ii_let_19940318_cairo-population-sadik_en.html.

———. "Letter to Women." June 29,1995. www.vatican.va/holy_father/john_paul_ii/letters/documents/hf_jp-ii_let_29061995_wo men_en.html.

———. "Maria Goretti: Example for Young People." *L'Osservatore Romano*, July 6, 2002. www.catholicculture.org/culture/library/view .cfm?id = 4414&repos = 1&subrepos = &searchid = 291002.

———. *Solicitudo rei socialis.* 1987.

———. *The Theology of the Body: Human Love in the Divine Plan.* Boston: Pauline Books and Media, 1997.

———. *Veritatis splendor* (*The Splendor of Truth*). 1993.

Jones, Serene. *Feminist Theory and Christian Theology: Cartographies of Grace.* Minneapolis: Fortress Press, 2000.

Jordan, Mark. *The Ethics of Sex.* Oxford: Blackwell, 2002.

———. *The Silence of Sodom.* Chicago: University of Chicago Press, 2000.

Jung, Patricia Beattie. "The Call to Wed: Why Catholics Should Cele-
brate Same-Sex Marriage." Dignity USA. www.dignityusa.org/pdf/
CallToWed-PBJ.pdf.

Kaczor, Christopher. *The Edge of Life: Human Dignity and Contemporary Bioethics.* Dordrecht: Springer, 2005.

———. "Proportionalism and the Pill: How Developments in Theory
Lead to Contradictions in Practice." *The Thomist* 63 (1999): 269–81.

Kalbian, Aline H. "Catholics and Contraception since 1968: Has Anything Really Changed?" *Louvain Studies* 36 (2012): 22–45.

———. *Sexing the Church: Gender, Power, and Ethics in Contemporary
Catholicism.* Bloomington: Indiana University Press, 2005.

Kaveny, M. Cathleen. "Appropriation of Evil: Cooperation's Mirror
Image." *Theological Studies* 61 (2000): 280–313.

———. "Intrinsic Evil and Political Responsibility." *America*, October
27, 2008.

———. *Law's Virtues: Fostering Autonomy and Solidarity in American
Society.* Washington, DC: Georgetown University Press, 2012.

Kaveny, M. Cathleen, and James F. Keenan. "Ethical Issues in Health-
Care Restructuring." *Theological Studies* 56, no. 1 (March 1995):
136–50.

Keenan, James F., SJ. "Applying the Seventeenth-Century Casuistry of
Accommodation to HIV Prevention." *Theological Studies* 60 (1999).

———, ed. *Catholic Ethicists on HIV/AIDS Prevention.* New York:
Continuum, 2000.

———. "Prophylactics, Toleration, and Cooperation: Contemporary
Problems and Traditional Principles." *International Philosophical
Quarterly* 28 (1988): 201–20.

Kellison, Rosemary. "Responsibility for the Just War: A Pragmatist-
Feminist Approach to the Study of Religious Ethics." PhD diss.,
2013.

Kelly, Kevin, MD. "AIDS and Ethics: An Overview." *General Hospital
Psychiatry* 9 (1987): 331–40.

Kelsay, John. "The Present State of the Comparative Study of Religious
Ethics: An Update." *Journal of Religious Ethics* 40, no. 4 (December
2012).

Kennedy, David M. *Birth Control in America: The Career of Margaret
Sanger.* New Haven, CT: Yale University Press, 1970.

Kowalewski, Mark R. "Religious Constructions of the AIDS Crisis."
*Sociological Analysis* 51, no. 1 (Spring 1990): 91–96.

Leo XIII, Pope. *Arcanum divinae sapientia* (*On Christian Marriage*). February 10, 1880. www.vatican.va/holy_father/leo_xiii/encyclicals/documents/hf_l-xiii_enc_10021880_arcanum_en.html.

———. *Syllabus of Errors.*

Lepani, Katherine. "Fitting Condoms on Culture: Rethinking Approaches to HIV Prevention in the Trobriand Islands, Papua New Guinea." In *Making Sense of AIDS: Culture, Sexuality, and Power in Melanesia*, edited by Leslie Butt and Richard Eves. Honolulu: University of Hawaii Press, 2008.

Lynch, John J., SJ. "Notes on Moral Theology." *Theological Studies* 23, no. 2 (June 1962).

Mahmood, Saba. *Politics of Piety: The Islamic Revival and the Feminist Subject.* Princeton, NJ: Princeton University Press, 2005.

Mahoney, John. *The Making of Moral Theology: A Study of the Roman Catholic Tradition.* Oxford: Clarendon Press, 1987.

Malthus, Thomas R. *An Essay on the Principle of Population.* London: Penguin, 1982.

Marchetto, Archbishop Agostino. *HIV/AIDS and Its Effects on Refugee Situations in a Christian Perspective.* Rome: Pontifical Council for the Pastoral Care of Migrants and Itinerant People, 2013. www.vatican.va/roman_curia/pontifical_councils/migrants/pom2006_101/rc_pc_migrants_pom101_hiv-aids.html.

May, William E. "Catholic Health Care and Contraception." *Ethics and Medics* 23, no. 5 (May 1998): 1–2.

McClory, Robert. *Turning Point: The Inside Story of the Papal Birth Control Comission, and How* Humanae vitae *Changed the Life of Patty Crowley and the Future of the Church.* New York: Crossroad, 1995.

McCormick, Richard A., SJ. "Anti-Fertility Pills." *Homiletic and Pastoral Review* 62, no. 8 (May 1962).

———. *The Critical Calling: Reflection on Moral Dilemmas since Vatican II.* Washington, DC: Georgetown University Press, 2006.

———. "Sterilization: The Dilemma of Catholic Hospitals." In *The Critical Calling: Reflections on Moral Dilemmas since Vatican II.* Washington, DC: Georgetown University Press, 1989.

McKenzie, Nancy F. *The AIDS Reader: Social, Political, and Ethical Issues.* New York: Meridian, Penguin Books, 1991.

Meassick, Elizabeth Onjoro. "HIV/AIDS Prevention: Strategies for Improving Prevention Efforts in Africa." In *AIDS, Culture, and*

*Africa*, edited by Douglas Feldman. Gainesville: University of Florida Press, 2008.

"Meeting of Catholic Organizations Engaged in the Response to HIV and AIDS." January 23–26, 2006. www.caritas.org/includes/pdf/GVAFinalRep.pdf.

Meilaender, Gilbert. "Sweet Necessities: Food, Sex, and St. Augustine." *Journal of Religious Ethics* 29, no. 1 (Spring 2001): 13–18.

Miller, Richard B. *Casuistry and Modern Ethics: A Poetics of Practical Reasoning.* Chicago: University of Chicago Press, 1993.

Murphy, Francis X. "Catholic Perspectives on Population Issues II." *Population Bulletin* 35, no. 6 (February 1981): 3–43.

Murphy, Patricia Aikins. "Update on Emergency Contraception." *Journal of Midwifery & Women's Health* 57, no. 6 (November–December 2012): 593–602.

National Conference of Catholic Bishops. *Called to Compassion and Responsibility: A Response to the HIV/AIDS Crisis.* 1989. http://old.usccb.org/sdwp/international/ctoresp.shtml#4.

National Conference of State Legislatures. "50-State Summary of Emergency Contraception Laws." www.ncsl.org/programs/health/ECleg.htm.

*New York Times.* "A World of Harm for Women." October 19, 2012.

Noonan, John T. *A Church That Can and Cannot Change: The Development of Catholic Moral Teaching.* Notre Dame, IN: University of Notre Dame Press, 2005.

———. *Contraception: A History of Its Treatment by the Catholic Theologians and Canonists.* Cambridge, MA: Harvard University Press, 1966.

Notare, T. "A Revolution in Christian Morals" (Resolution 15 of Lambeth 1930). *Revue d'Histoire Ecclesiastique* 94 (April 1999): 471–501.

"Notification of the Congregation for the Doctrine of the Faith regarding the Book *Just Love: A Framework for Christian Sexual Ethics* by Sister Margaret A. Farley, RSM." April 6, 2012. http://press.catholica.va/news_services/bulletin/news/29292.php?index=29292&lang=en#.

Odozor, Paulinus. *Moral Theology in an Age of Renewal: A Study of the Catholic Tradition since Vatican II.* Notre Dame, IN: University of Notre Dame Press, 2003.

Office of Population Affairs, US Department of Health and Human Services. "Emergency Contraception Fact Sheet." www.hhs.gov/opa/pdfs/emergency-contraception-fact-sheet.pdf.

O'Malley, John W. "'The Hermeneutic of Reform': A Historical Analysis." *Theological Studies* 73, no. 3 (2012): 517–46.

———. *What Happened at Vatican II.* Cambridge, MA: Belknap Press of Harvard University Press, 2009.

Omer, Atalia. "Rejoinder: On Professor McCutcheon's (Un)Critical Caretaking." *Journal of the American Academy of Religion* 80, no. 4 (2012): 1084–85.

Patrick, Anne. "Narrative and the Social Dynamics of Virtue." In *Virtue: Readings in Moral Theology No. 16*, edited by Charles E. Curran and Lisa A. Fullam. New York: Paulist Press, 2011.

Paul VI, Pope. *Humanae vitae.* 1968.

———. *Populorum progressio.* 1967.

Pinckaers, Servais. *Morality: The Catholic View*, edited and translated by Michael Sherwin, OP. South Bend, IN: Saint Augustine's Press, 2001.

Pius XI, Pope. *Casti connubii.* 1930.

Pollack, Andrew, and Donald G. McNeil Jr. "In Medical First, a Baby with HIV Is Deemed Cured." *New York Times*, March 3, 2013. www.nytimes.com/2013/03/04/health/for-first-time-baby-cured-of-hiv-doctors-say.html?pagewanted=all&_r=0.

Pontifical Academy for Life. "Final Declaration by the 13th General Assembly and the International Congress on 'The Christian Conscience in Support of the Right to Life.'" March 15, 2007. www.vati can.va/roman_curia/pontifical_academies/acdlife/documents/rc_ pont-acd_life_doc_20070315_xiii-gen-assembly-final_en.html.

———. "Statement on the So-Called 'Morning-After Pill.'" October 31, 2000. www.vatican.va/roman_curia/pontifical_academies/acd life/documents/rc_pa_acdlife_doc_20001031_pillola-giorno-dopo _en.html.

Porter, Jean. *Natural and Divine Law: Reclaiming the Tradition for Christian Ethics.* Grand Rapids: Eerdmans, 1999.

Ramsey, Paul. "Human Sexuality in the History of Redemption." *Journal of Religious Ethics* 16, no. 1 (Spring 1988): 56–86.

Rao, Mohan, and Sarah Sexton. "Introduction: Population, Health, and Gender in Neo-Liberal Times." In *Markets and Malthus: Population, Gender, and Health in Neo-Liberal Times*, edited by Mohan Rao and Sarah Sexton. New Delhi: Sage, 2010.

Ratzinger, Joseph Cardinal. *Instruction on the Ecclesial Vocation of the Theologian.* May 24, 1990. www.ewtn.com/library/curia/cdftheo .htm.

Rhonheimer, Martin. *Ethics of Procreation & the Defense of Human Life: Contraception, Artificial Fertilization, and Abortion.* Washington, DC: Catholic University of America Press, 2010.

Riddle, John M. *Contraception and Abortion from the Ancient World to the Renaissance.* Cambridge, MA: Harvard University Press, 1994.

Riedemann, Mark. "An African View of Church and HIV: Interview with Founder of Nairobi-Based AIDS Network." *Zenit,* November 29, 2010. Originally conducted for *Where God Weeps,* produced by Catholic Radio and Television Network.

Roberts, Dorothy. *Killing the Black Body: Race, Reproduction, and the Meaning of Liberty.* New York: Vintage Books, 1997.

Rock, John. "We Can End the Battle over Birth Control." *Good Housekeeping,* July 1961, 107–10.

Rodlach, Alexander. *Witches, Westerners, and HIV: AIDS & Cultures of Blame in Africa.* Walnut Grove, CA: Left Coast Press, 2006.

Rubio, Julie Hanlon. "Beyond the Liberal/Conservative Divide on Contraception: The Wisdom of Practitioners of Natural Family Planning and Artificial Birth Control." *Horizons* 32, no. 3 (2005): 270–94.

Ryan, John. *Family Limitation and the Church and Birth Control.* New York: Paulist Press, 1916.

Sabia, Dan. "Defending Immanent Critique." *Political Theory* 38, no. 5 (2010): 684–711.

Salzman, Todd A., and Michael G. Lawler. *The Sexual Person: Toward a Renewed Catholic Anthropology.* Washington, DC: Georgetown University Press, 2008.

Sanfilippo, Joseph, and Don Downing. "Emergency Contraception: When and How to Use It." *Journal of Family Practice,* February 2008.

Sanger, Margaret. *The Pivot of Civilization.* New York: Brentano's, 1922.

Schoepf, Brooke G. "Uganda: Lessons for AIDS Control in Africa." *Review of African Political Economy* 98 (2003): 553–72.

Schulenburg, Jane Tibbetts. *Forgetful of Their Sex: Female Sanctity and Society ca. 500–1100.* Chicago: University of Chicago Press, 1998.

Scott, Joan W. "Gender: A Useful Category of Historical Analysis." *American Historical Review* 91, no. 5 (December 1986): 1053–75.

Second Vatican Council. *Dignitatis humanae (Declaration on Religious Freedom).* In *The Documents of Vatican II,* edited by Walter M. Abbott. New York: America Press, 1966.

———. *Gaudium et spes* (*The Church in the Modern World*). In *Catholic Social Thought: The Documentary Heritage*, edited by David J. O'Brien and Thomas A. Shannon. Maryknoll, NY: Orbis Press, 1992.

———. *Lumen gentium* (*Dogmatic Constitution on the Church*). In *The Documents of Vatican II*, edited by Walter M. Abbott. New York: America Press, 1966.

———. *Optatum totius* (*Decree on Priestly Formation*). In *The Documents of Vatican II*, edited by Walter M. Abbott. New York: America Press, 1966.

Selling, Joseph A. "Magisterial Teaching on Marriage 1880–1986: Historical Constancy or Radical Development?" In *Dialogue about Catholic Sexual Teaching*, edited by Charles E. Curran and Richard A. McCormick, SJ. New York: Paulist Press, 1993.

Sinding, Steven W. "Does 'CNN' (Condoms, Needles, Negotiation) Work Better than 'ABC' (Abstinence, Being Faithful, and Condom Use) in Attacking the AIDS Epidemic?" *International Family Planning Perspectives* 31, no. 1 (March 2005): 38–40.

Slutkin, Gary, Sam Okware, Warren Naamara, Don Sutherland, Donna Flanagan, Michel Carael, Erik Blas, Paul Delay, and Daniel Tarantola. "How Uganda Reversed Its HIV Epidemic." *AIDS Behavior* 10 (2006): 351–56.

Spadaro, Antonio, SJ. "A Big Heart Open to God: The Exclusive Interview with Pope Francis." *America*, September 30, 2013: 15–38.

St. John-Stevas, Norman. *The Agonising Choice: Birth Control, Religion, and Law.* London: Eyre & Spottiswoode, 1971.

"Statement by Catholic Theologians, Washington, DC, July 30, 1968." In *Dialogue about Sexual Teaching*, edited by Charles E. Curran and Richard A. McCormick. New York: Paulist Press, 1993.

Stout, Jeffrey. "Commitments and Traditions in the Study of Religious Ethics." *Journal of Religious Ethics* 25, no. 3 (25th Anniversary Supplement, 1998): 23–56.

Sullivan, Francis A., SJ. "Development in Teaching Authority since Vatican II." *Theological Studies* 73, no. 3 (2012): 570–89.

———. *Magisterium: Teaching Authority in the Catholic Church.* New York: Paulist Press, 1983.

Sulmasy, Daniel P. "Catholic Participation in Needle- and Syringe-Exchange Programs for Injection-Drug Users: An Ethical Analysis." *Theological Studies* 73 (2012): 422–41.

———. "Emergency Contraception for Women Who Have Been Raped: Must Catholics Test for Ovulation, or Is Testing for Pregnancy Morally Sufficient?" *Kennedy Institute of Ethics Journal* 16, no. 4 (2006).

Swanson, Karna. "Beyond Condoms in the AIDS Debate: Interview with Caritas Expert on HIV." *Zenit*, July 31, 2008. www.zenit.org/article-23393?!=english.

Symposium of Episcopal Conferences of Africa and Madagascar. "The Church in Africa in the Face of the HIV/AIDS Pandemic: Our Prayer Is Always Full of Hope." www.mission-preciousblood.org/Justice/Church_in_Africa_vs_HIV.doc.

Tentler, Leslie Woodcock. *Catholics and Contraception: An American History*. Ithaca, NY: Cornell University Press, 2004.

Tonti-Filippini, Nicholas, and Mary Walsh. "Postcoital Intervention: From Fear of Pregnancy to Rape Crisis." *National Catholic Bioethics Quarterly* 4, no. 2 (Summer 2004): 275–88.

Trujillo, Alfonso Cardinal López. "Family Values versus Safe Sex." December 1, 2003. www.vatican.va/roman_curia/pontifical_councils/family/documents/rc_pc_family_doc_20031201_family-values-safe-sex-trujillo_en.html#ChurchCriticism.

UNAIDS. "Condoms and HIV Prevention: Position Statement by UNAIDS, UNFPA and WHO." March 19, 2009. www.unaids.org/en/resources/presscentre/featurestories/2009/march /20090319prevention position.

United Nations, Department of Economic and Social Affairs, Population Division. *World Population Prospects: The 2010 Revision*, CD-ROM ed. 2011.

US Conference of Catholic Bishops. "Bishops' Pro-Life Chair Strongly Opposes Recommended Mandate for Birth Control Sterilization in Private Health Plans." July 19, 2011. http://old.usccb.org/comm/archives/2011/11–143.shtml.

———. "Bishops Urge Congress to Make the Poor a Priority in Economic Recovery Legislation." January 29, 2009. www.usccb.org/comm/archives/2009/09–026.shtml.

———. *Ethical and Religious Directives for Catholic Health Care Services*, 5th ed. Washington, DC: US Conference of Catholic Bishops, 2009. www.usccb.org/issues-and-action/human-life-and-dignity/health-care/upload/Ethical-Religious-Directives-Catholic-Health-Care-Services-fifth-edition-2009.pdf.

———. "HHS Mandate for Contraceptive and Abortifacient Drugs Violates Conscience Rights." August 1, 2011. www.usccb.org/news/2011/11–154.cfm.

———. *The Many Faces of AIDS: A Gospel Response. Origins* 17, no. 28 (1987): 482–89. http://old.usccb.org/sdwp/international/mfa87.shtml.

———. *Pastoral Letter of 1919.* www.ewtn.com/library/bishops/PL1919.htm.

———. "Questions and Answers about HIV/AIDS." www.usccb.org/comm/q&aabouthiv-aids.pdf.

———. "USCCB Says Administration Mandate Violates First Amendment Freedom of Religious Organizations and Others." March 20, 2013. www.usccb.org/news/2013/13–054.cfm.

Valsecchi, Ambrogio. *Controversy: The Birth Control Debate 1958–1968,* translated by Dorothy White. Washington, DC: Corpus Books, 1968.

Vatican. "Statement of Interpretation of the Holy See on the Adoption of the Declaration of Commitment on HIV/AIDS." June 27, 2001. www.vatican.va/roman_curia/secratariat_state/documents/rc_seg-st_doc_20010627.

Vitillo, Robert J. *Action in Response to HIV Pandemic 2003–2007.* Report to Eighteenth General Assembly of Caritas Internationalis, April 9, 2007.

von Hertzen, Helena, and Paul F. A. Van Look. "Research on New Methods of Emergency Contraception." *Family Planning Perspectives* 28, no. 2 (March–April 1996).

Walker, Margaret Urban. *Moral Understandings: A Feminist Study of Ethics,* 2nd ed. Oxford: Oxford University Press, 2007.

Warner, L., K. M. Stone, M. Macaluso, J. W. Buehler, and H. D. Austin. "Condom Use and Risk of Gonorrhea and Chlamydia: A Systematic Review of Design and Measurement Factors Assessed in Epidemiologic Studies." *Sexually Transmitted Disease* 33, no. 1 (January 2006): 36–51.

Watkins, Elizabeth S. *On the Pill: A Social History of Oral Contraceptives, 1950–1970.* Baltimore: Johns Hopkins University Press, 1998.

Weigel, George. "What Really Happened at Cairo?" *First Things,* February 1995, 24–31.

Wojtyla, Karol (John Paul II). *Love and Responsibility,* rev. ed. San Francisco: Ignatius Press, 1993.

Wood, Alastair J. J., Jeffrey M. Drazen, and Michael F. Greene. "The Politics of Emergency Contraception." *New England Journal of Medicine* 366, no. 2 (January 12, 2012): 101–2.

Zlidar, V. M., R. Gardner, S. O. Rutstein, L. Morris, H. Goldberg, and K. Johnson. *New Survey Findings: The Reproductive Revolution Continues—Population Reports*. INFO Project, series M, no. 17. Baltimore: Johns Hopkins Bloomberg School of Public Health, 2003. www.infoforhealth.org/pr/m17/.

Zuger, Abigail. "AIDS on the Wards; A Residency in Medical Ethics." *Hastings Center Report* 17, no. 3 (June 1987): 16–20.

# INDEX

ABC model for HIV/AIDS prevention,
69–70

abortion: Augustine on, 39; and Cairo
Conference (1994), 160; early
Christian opposition to, 41–44,
57n43; emergency contraception
and concerns about, 21, 96, 99–100,
101–3; and the Fifth
Commandment, 16–17, 20–22,
26n39; John Paul II on contraception and, 17, 26n39; John Paul II
on rape and, 115; and magic, 43;
persistent association of contraception and, 17, 21, 99–100, 101–3;
population and development issues,
137–38, 160; *Roe v. Wade* decision,
137; Roman (pagan) practices,
41–44, 57n43, 103; and US policies
on international family planning,
137–38

abstinence-based HIV prevention
programs, 69–70, 71–73

adultery: and the *Catechism*, 16, 22–23;
as failure in chastity, 26n38; Jesus
on, 22; Sixth Commandment, 16,
22–23, 79. *See also* marital sexuality

Africa, Sub-Saharan: Catholic anticondom messages and local cultural
views of procreation, 69; Catholic
charities and HIV/AIDS, 67–68;
HIV/AIDS infection and transmission rates, 64–65, 91nn16–17

Albert, Saint, 43

Anglican Church, 34

Anwarite, Saint Marie Clementine,
128n71

Aquinas, Thomas: on contraception
and the preservation of the species,
17, 26n40; on contraception as sin
against nature, 32–33; on the Decalogue and natural law, 18–19;
definition of rape and sins of lust,
113–14, 128n61; natural law arguments about procreative purpose of
sexual act, 32–33, 42, 44, 52; and
Ryan's explication of the Catholic
position on birth control, 152;
*Summa Theologiae*, 18–19, 32–33

Athenagoras, 57n43

Augustine of Hippo, Saint: on abortion,
39; *Confessions*, 38–40; on contraception and sexuality in marriage,
38–40, 42; discussion of contraception (the *Aliquando*), 39–40; on
infanticide, 39; on rape and the
victim's purity, 116–17; on remarriage after divorce, 39–40; and sin of
Onan, 40, 56n22; on threefold
purpose of marriage, 39

Barragán, Javier Cardinal Lozano,
78–79

Bayer, Edward, 109–11, 117, 127n41

Benedict XVI, Pope: *Caritatis in
veritate*, 146–48; contraception and
social justice, 146–48; *Light of the
World* interview (2010), 75; and Paul
VI's *Populorum progressio*, 146;
population and "integral development," 146–48; statements about
condoms for HIV/AIDS
prevention, 74–75, 92n53; statements on the HIV/AIDS epidemic,
74–75, 92n53; theological anthropology and dignity of the human
person, 78; on vocation of the theologian, 82